Zebrafish in Biomedical Research

Edited by Yusuf Bozkurt

Published in London, United Kingdom

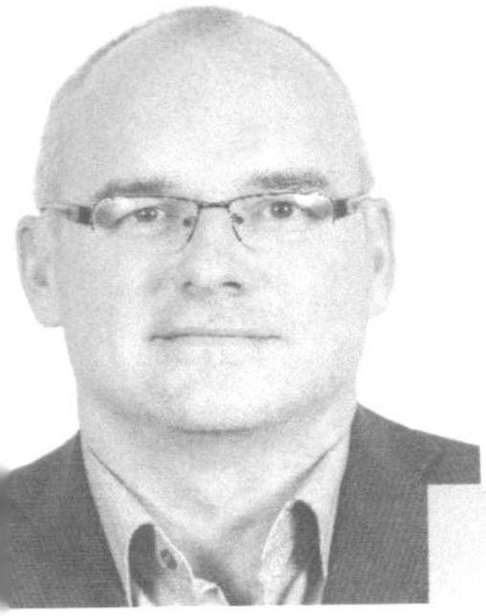
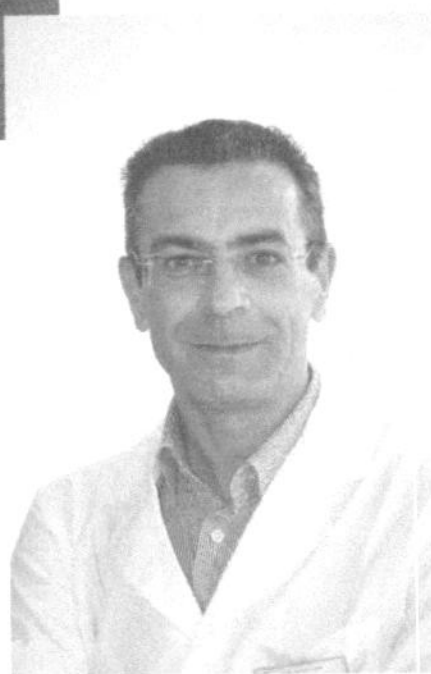
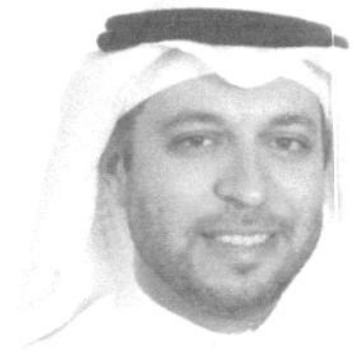
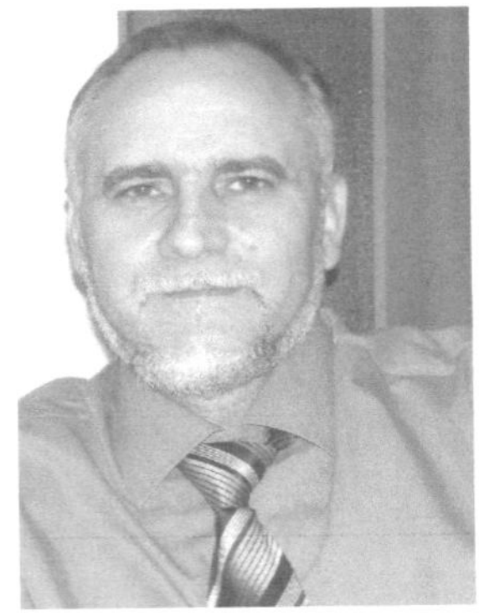
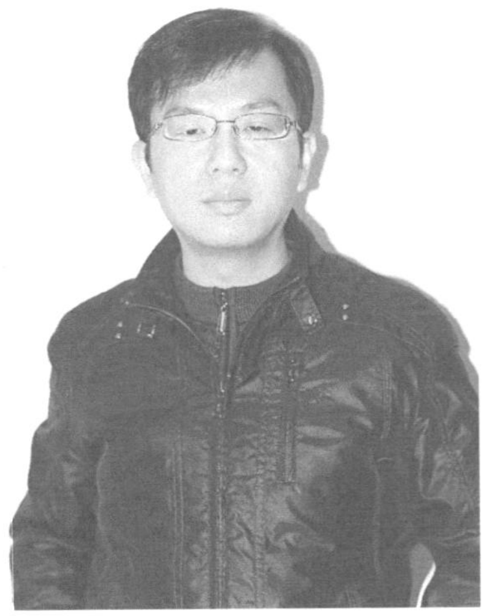
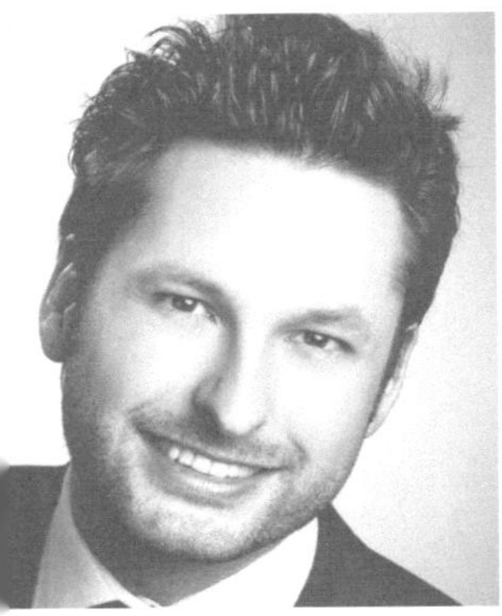
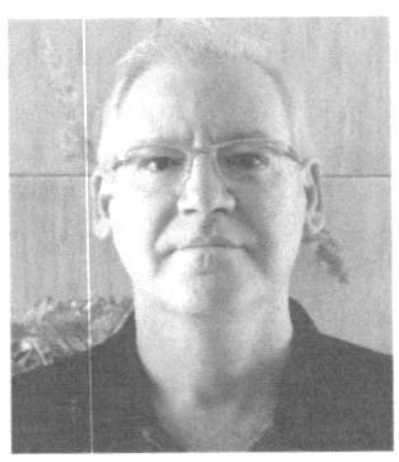

IntechOpen

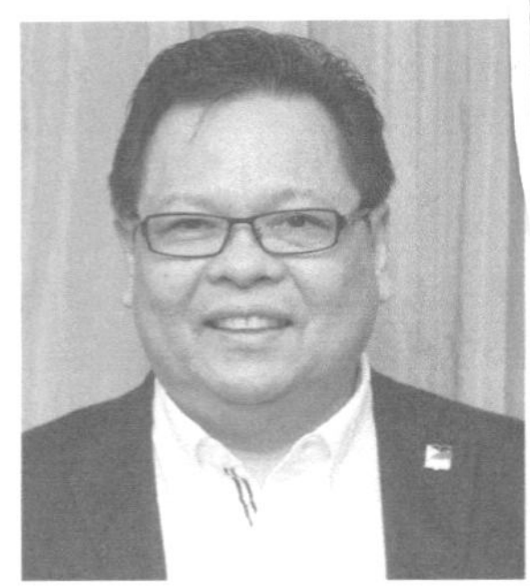
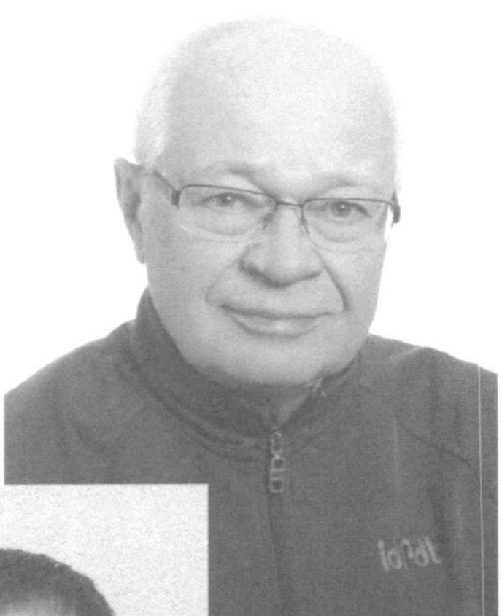
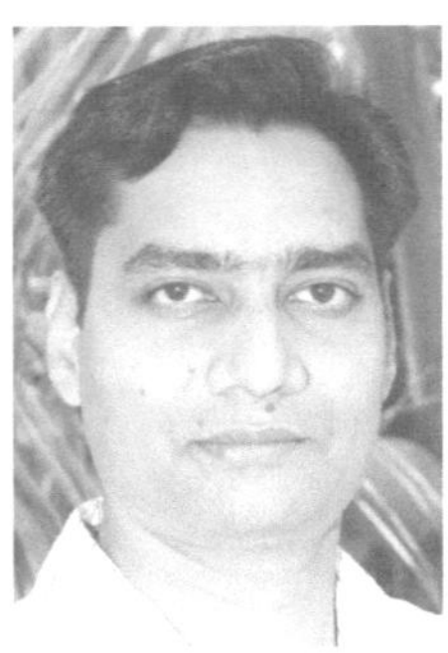
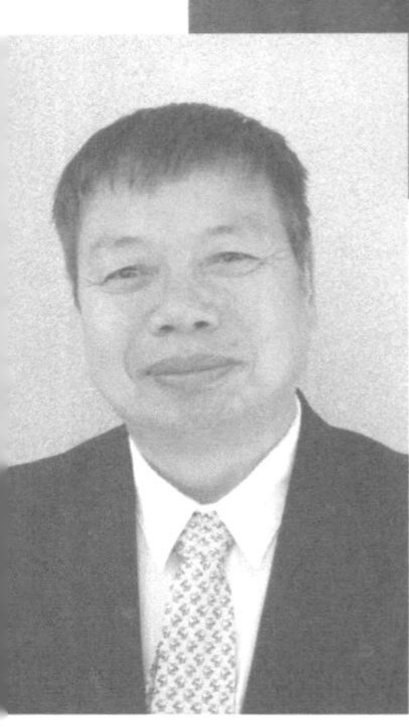
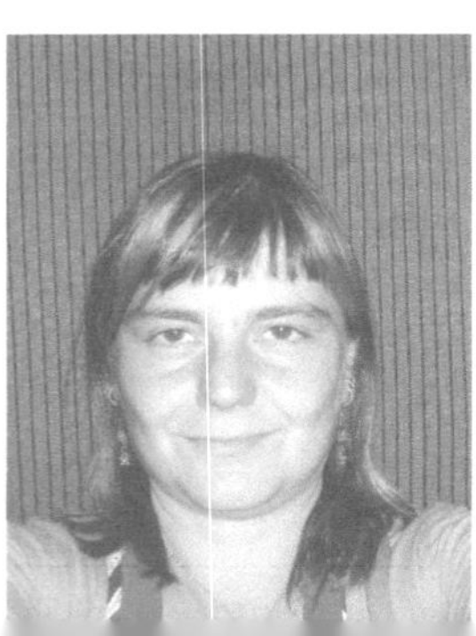
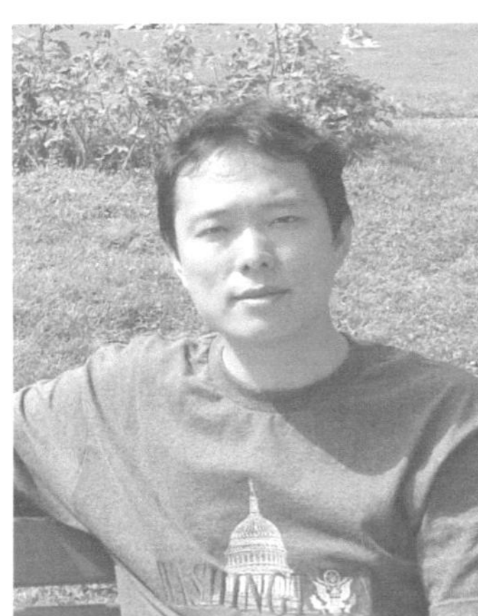

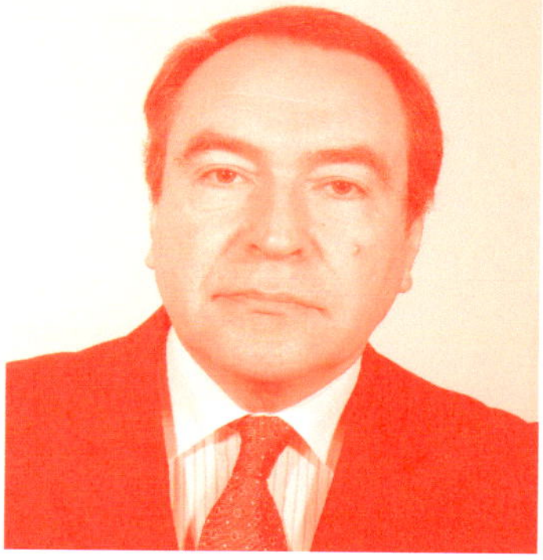
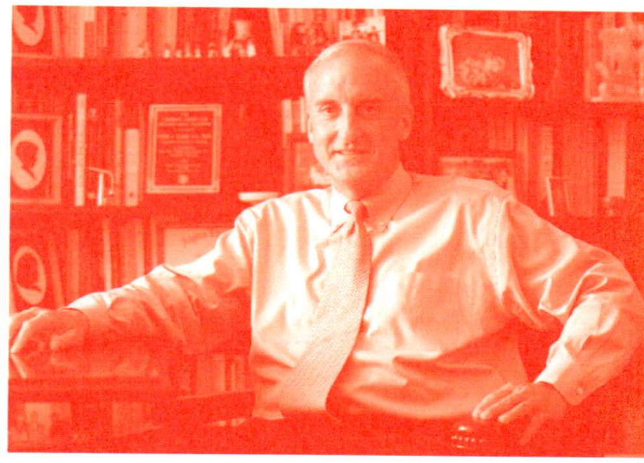
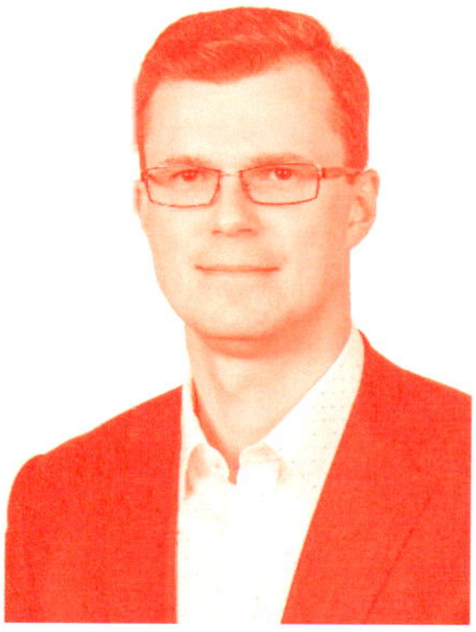
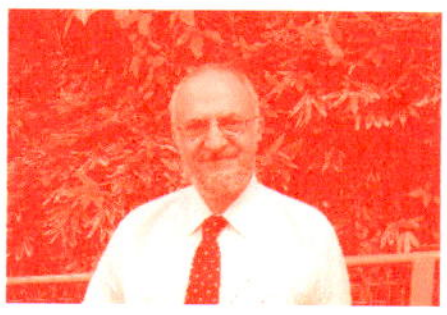
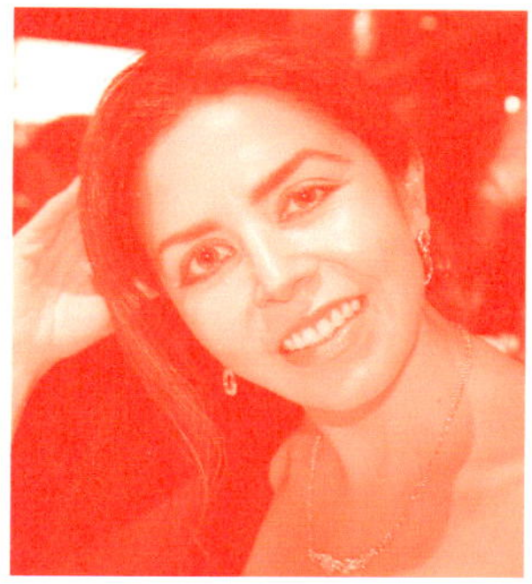

Supporting open minds since 2005

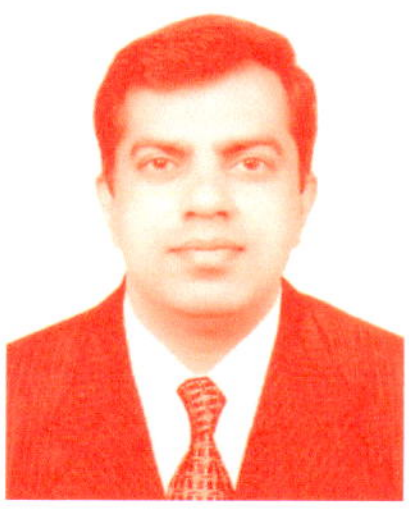
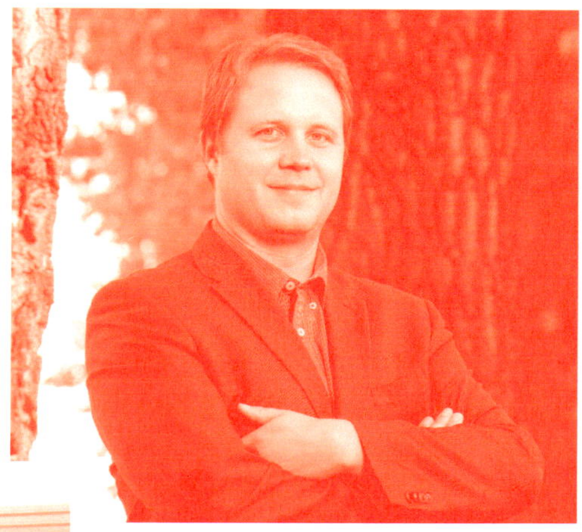
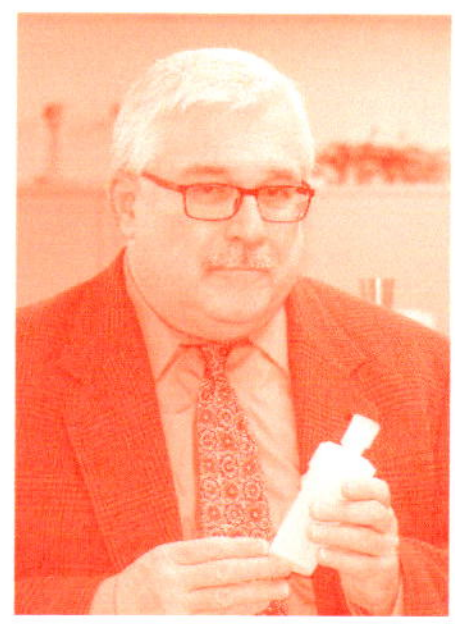
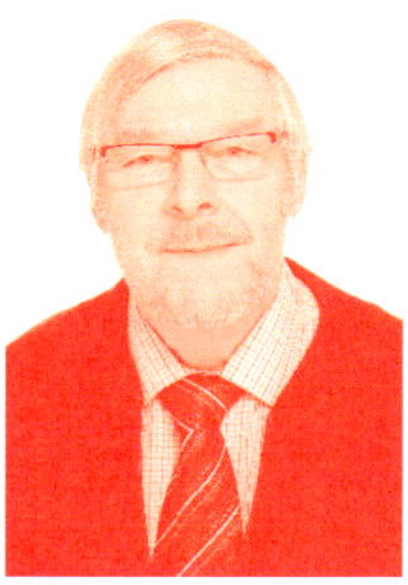
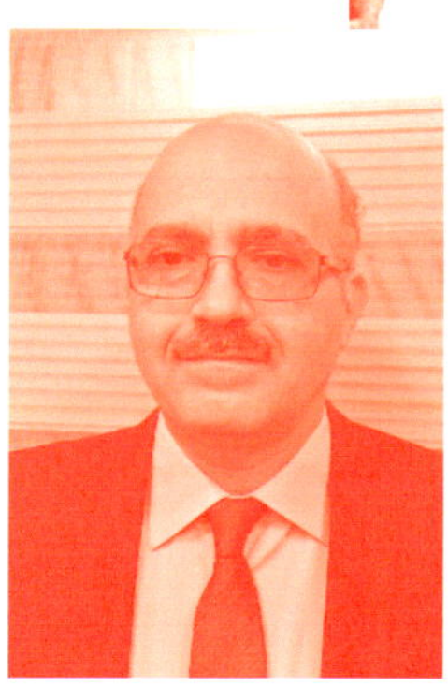
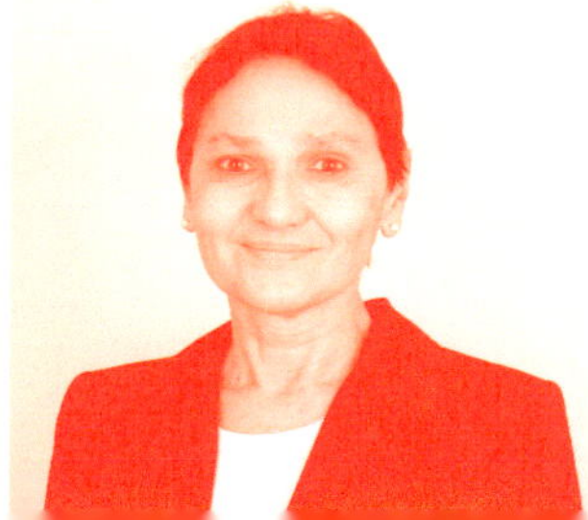
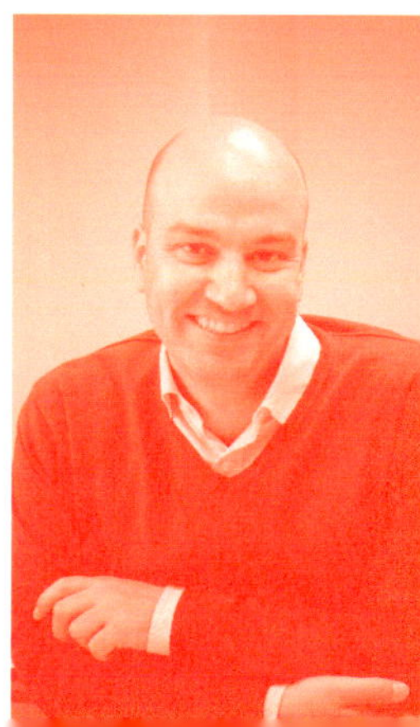

Zebrafish in Biomedical Research
http://dx.doi.org/10.5772/intechopen.82977
Edited by Yusuf Bozkurt

Contributors
Mónica Roxo-Rosa, Susana S. Lopes, José Carlos Tavares Carvalho, Luis David Solis Murgas, Ruchi Jakhmola-Mani, Deepshikha Pande Katare, Khyati Mittal, Yusuf Bozkurt

First published in London, United Kingdom, 2020 by IntechOpen
IntechOpen is the global imprint of INTECHOPEN LIMITED, registered in England and Wales, registration number: 11086078, 7th floor, 10 Lower Thames Street, London, EC3R 6AF, United Kingdom
Printed in Croatia

British Library Cataloguing-in-Publication Data
A catalogue record for this book is available from the British Library

Additional hard and PDF copies can be obtained from orders@intechopen.com

Zebrafish in Biomedical Research
Edited by Yusuf Bozkurt
p. cm.
Print ISBN 978-1-78985-985-0
Online ISBN 978-1-78985-986-7
eBook (PDF) ISBN 978-1-78985-573-9

Meet the editor

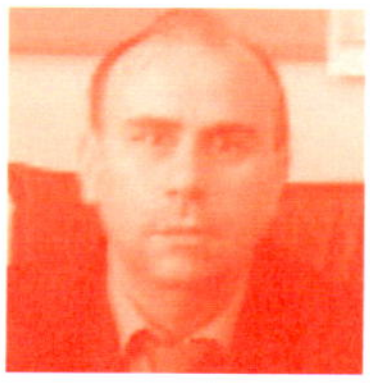

Yusuf Bozkurt holds a BSc, MSc, and PhD from Ankara University (Turkey). He is currently Professor of Biotechnology of Reproduction in the field of Aquaculture at İskenderun Technical University (Turkey). His research interests include reproductive biology and biotechnology with an emphasis on cryopreservation. Dr. Bozkurt has studied in Spain and Hungary and has authored many research articles published in indexed journals and books. Also, he has participated in many international and national congresses, seminars and workshops with oral and poster presentations. He is currently a member of the European Aquaculture society (EAS).

Contents

Preface

In recent years, the zebrafish has become a favorite model organism in biomedical research in order to understand and treat certain health problems such as cancer and some genetic and neurological disorders. Among its various advantages, the zebrafish has a transparent embryo, which allows visualization of development and morphogenesis of its tissues and organs. This is very important in understanding the different mechanisms underlying health problems.

Zebrafish in Biomedical Research describes the current understanding of zebrafish as a model organism in biomedical science. This book is divided into five chapters over four sections as follows.

Section 1, "Zebrafish: A Model Organism," is an introductory section including Chapter 1, "Importance of Zebrafish (*Danio rerio*) as a Model Organism in Biomedical Research." This chapter focusses on recent developments in using zebrafish in research to examine the different mechanisms underlying human health problems.

Section 2, "Using of Zebrafish in Neurological Studies," includes Chapter 2, "Alarm Test: A Novel Chemical Free Behaviour Assesment Tool for Zebrafish." This chapter provides valuable information regarding using zebrafish as an animal model for understanding and treating some neurological diseases such as Alzheimer's and Parkinson's. It describes an alarm test that measures anxiety level and stress response in zebrafish kept in isolated and herd conditions.

Section 3, "Using of Zebrafish in Miscellaneous Diseases," is divided into two chapters. Chapter 3, "The Zebrafish Kupffer's Vesicle: A Special Organ in a Model Organism to Study Human Diseases," examines the underlying mechanisms and problems of both Primary Ciliary Dyskinesia (PCD) and Autosomal Dominant Polycystic Kidney Disease (ADPKD) via the (Kupffer's Vesicle) KV, which is an organ transiently present in the early embryonic life of the zebrafish. Chapter 4, "Zebrafish as an Experimental Model for the Study of Obesity," discusses using zebrafish to examine the physiological mechanisms of obesity and related metabolic disorders, such as cardiovascular dysfunction, diabetes and cancer.

Section 4, "Using of Zebrafish in Toxicology and Drug Development" includes Chapter 5, "Histopathology of Zebrafish (*Danio rerio*) in Non-Clinical Toxicological Studies of New Drugs." This chapter researches the effect of environmental toxicity on different major organs of zebrafish, such as gills, kidney, liver and intestines, via examining healthy and damaged histopathology of these organs.

I would like to thank all the authors for their distinguished contributions, IntechOpen Publishing, and its Author Service Manager Ms. Jasna Bozic for her help in preparing this book for publication.

Yusuf Bozkurt
Professor,
Faculty of Marine Sciences and Technology,
İskenderun Technical University,
İskenderun, Hatay, Turkey

Section 1

Zebrafish: A Model Organism

Chapter 1

Introductory Chapter: Importance of Zebrafish (*Danio rerio*) as Model Organism in Biomedical Research

Yusuf Bozkurt

1. Introduction

Animal experimentation has an important role in scientific research. Although some models have been replaced by alternative methods, scientific research still needs animal models for development, reliability, and legitimacy of science [1].

From this point of view, biomedical research relies on using of animal models in order to understand a particular disease without causing risk to the human being [2]. On the other hand, as it is known, research costs are high especially carried out with mammals. Therefore, a new model of animal experiments, including invertebrates and fish species, becomes necessary recently. Thus, as a result of searching new experimental models, in order to reduce cost and save time, the zebrafish was discovered.

As a result, using of zebrafish (*Danio rerio*), which is one of the tropical freshwater fish species, has increased its importance as an experimental animal model in the field of biomedical research in recent years.

2. The zebrafish (*Danio rerio*)

The zebrafish belongs to the *Cyprinidae* family, which consists of more than 2000 species [3]. Its former scientific name was *Brachydanio rerio*, but it was changed to *Danio rerio* in 1981 [4], because both genera were very similar by having short dorsal fins and absent or incomplete lateral lines [5].

Zebrafish is a small tropical freshwater fish which lives in river basins of India, Northern Pakistan, Nepal, Bhutan, and South Asia. Their maturation period takes only 2–3 months, which is relatively less laborious and time-saving for generating of transgenic lines. Zebrafish can produce 200–300 fertilized eggs weekly and complete the embryogenesis in 72 h. Pigmentation in the embryos starts about 30–72 h postfertilization [6].

Its adults are about 2.5–4 cm long, and its larval stage is transparent. On the other hand, when it has reached the adult stage, it develops a stripe along with the length of the body, and it looks blue in color. Males are slender and torpedo-shaped, usually with a pink or yellow color.

3. Advantages of zebrafish usage in biomedical research

Although zebrafish (*Danio rerio*) is a primitive vertebrate, it has several advantages over other model organisms. The main reasons for it becoming an excellent model organism in different research fields are easy access to all stages of its body development, transparency of its embryos and larvaes, high genetic similarity, and homologous physiology with human beings especially in terms of the central nervous system.

Besides these, adults and embryos of this species are small in size and have a lower cost, and the generation interval is short. Furthermore, they show rapid development and hatches in less than 3 days and become mature in 90 days which the search more rapid [7].

Additionally, microinjection of fertilized eggs is easily accessible and relatively cheap. The embryos of zebrafish develop outside the mother's body and are transparent. The transparency of the zebrafish embryo facilitates the studies in genetic development programs, because it is possible to monitor and manipulate its development without difficulties. Interestingly, the morphology of the brain of mammals and zebrafish is similar, including macro-organization of the brain [7].

Furthermore, their genome sizes are approximately 20–40% of the mammalian genome, and it makes them the only vertebrates available for large-scale mutagenesis. In addition, many routine techniques of molecular biology and genetics, including knock-in, knockdown, and knockout, are well developed in the zebrafish [8].

4. Studies carried out with zebrafish in biomedical research

4.1 Hematopoetical research

Zebrafish play an important role in the study of hematopoiesis. Because these fishes have the same sequential multilineage hematopoiesis process as human beings, these model organisms provide many insights, both in blood lineage development pathways and blood disorders, to the scientists who are studying in the field of medicine [9].

4.2 Cardiovascular research

These fishes are also largely used to explore cardiovascular disorders since they have a similar embryonic heart structure as that of human embryos. Furthermore, zebrafish have the advantage of being able to survive without adequate cardiac circulation. The excellent feature helps the embryo which develops from the initial phases despite cardiovascular defects. For instance, one of the patterns of their use within this field is exploration of the link between inflammation and myocardial infarction [9].

4.3 Cryobiological research

The small size and good fecundity of the zebrafish make it suitable for the cryobiological and genetic studies. However, limited animal facility space and the need to maintain broodstock lines are important restraining factors for the researches carried out with zebrafish [10, 11].

Cryopreservation is the process of freezing the biological material at a temperature of liquid nitrogen (LN_2) (−196°C). This means biological activities discontinue including the biochemical reactions creating cell death and DNA damage at these low temperatures [12]. In this way, it is possible to store the biological materials unchanged for centuries with the capability of recovering the cell functionality following the thawing process [13].

From this point of view, efficient sperm cryopreservation procedure can help overcome these problems by reducing the number of live fish in a system while maintaining their reproductive capacity [12, 14]. Sperm cryopreservation also provides "genetic insurance" for the recovery of strains in case the living stocks are lost [15, 16] and extends the functional reproductive lifetime of males as long as samples maintain viable in storage [17]. Finally, the technique has been utilized in reverse-genetic mutagenesis approaches, in which a cryopreserved sperm library is used to recover heterozygote mutant fish of interest [18]. Thus, an optimized zebrafish sperm cryopreservation protocol will not only increase the efficacy of this genetic screening method but also benefit the zebrafish community as a whole.

4.4 Neurological research

Another important research field is the curing of neurological disorders with the zebrafish because of the abundance of the same signaling proteins in the brains of human beings. It is also known that several human neurological disorders have also an equivalent in the zebrafish [7].

4.5 Aquaculture research

Zebrafish is also one of the genetically more malleable aquatic species among different fish species in aquaculture. The zebrafish model is used commercially in many areas of aquaculture such as in the identification of genes involved in the development of the muscles, bones, and fats, metabolism of the nutrients, disease and stress pathways, and also behavioral traits.

The drugs affecting the physiology of the fishes can easily be tested in zebrafish especially in terms of their effect on a range of alleles in order to determine their genetic property [19]. Additionally, many researches have been done regarding improvement of diet and their husbandry to improve growth rate and reduce stress and disease in many fish species.

5. Conclusion

It can be concluded that zebrafish is a successful and versatile animal, offering a tool to model regarding gene function, development of various organ systems, cancer studies, toxicology, drug discovery, human disease and disorders, and also aquaculture.

The usefulness of zebrafish has excelled in biomedical research because of its low cost and easy maintenance, transparent embryo, easy manipulation, high fecundity, and rapid embryonic development.

From this point of view, the future of zebrafish as a model organism is very bright. In the coming years, an increased number of reports are expected on the application of zebrafish as an effective bioindicator. On the other hand, there is still much to discover about this species, and also it is necessary to put more efforts so that new information can flow to the understanding of biomedical research combined with the use of zebrafish.

Author details

Yusuf Bozkurt
Faculty of Marine Sciences and Technology, İskenderun Technical University, İskenderun, Hatay, Turkey

*Address all correspondence to: yfbozkurt@hotmail.com

References

[1] Simonetti RB, Marques LS, Streit DP Jr, Oberst ER. Journal of Fisheries Sciences. 2015;**9**(3):39-45

[2] Lieschke GJ, Currie PD. Animal models of human disease: Zebrafish swim into view. Nature Reviews. 2007;**8**:353-367

[3] Available from: http://www.fishbase.org/Summary/SpeciesSummary.php?ID=4653&AT=zebrafish [Accessed: 06 January 2020]

[4] Chu XL. A preliminary revision of fishes of the genus *Danio* from China. Zoology Research. 1981;**2**:145-156

[5] Fang F. Phylogenetic analysis of the Asian cyprinid genus *Danio* (Teleostei, Cyprinidae). Copeia. 2003;**52**:714-728

[6] Hill AJ, Teraoka H, Heideman W, Peterson RE. Zebrafish as a model vertebrate for investigating chemical toxicity: Review. Toxicological Science. 2005;**86**(1):6-19

[7] Kalueff AV, Stewart AM, Gerlai R. Zebrafish as an emerging model for studying complex brain disorders. Trends in Pharmacological Sciences. 2013;**35**(2):63-75

[8] Lantz-Mcpeak S, Guo X, Cuevas E, et al. Developmental toxicity assay using high content screening of zebrafish embryos. Journal of Applied Toxicology. 2014;**35**(3):261-272

[9] Available from: https://www.news-medical.net/life-sciences/Zebrafish-as-a Model-Organism.aspx [Accessed: 06 January 2020]

[10] Brand M, Granato M, Nusslein-Volhard C. Keeping and raising zebrafish. In: Nusslein-Volhard C, Dahm R, editors. Zebrafish: A Practical Approach. New York: Oxford University Press; 2002. pp. 7-37

[11] Westerfield M. The Zebrafish Book: A Guide for the Laboratory Use of Zebrafish (*Danio rerio*). Eugene, OR: University of Oregon Press; 2000

[12] Bozkurt Y, Yavaş İ, Gül A, Bucak MN, Yeni D, Avdatek F. Effect of extender supplemented with boron on post-thaw motility, viability, DNA damage and fertilization ability of cryopreserved brown trout (*Salmo trutta macrostigma*) spermatozoa. CryoLetters. 2019a;**40**(5):275-283

[13] Bozkurt Y. Introductory chapter: Application fields of cryopreservation biotechnology. In: Bozkurt Y, editor. Cryopreservation Biotechnology in Biomedical and Biological Sciences, Section I. London, United Kingdom: IntechOpen; 2018. pp. 1-4. ISBN: 978-1-78984-680-5

[14] Bozkurt Y. Introductory chapter: Cryopreservation biotechnology in aquatic science. In: Bozkurt Y, editor. Biological Research in Aquatic Science, Section I. London, United Kingdom: IntechOpen; 2019. pp. 3-8. ISBN: 978-1-78923-813-6

[15] Bozkurt Y, Yavaş İ, Bucak MN, Yeni D. Effect of different cryoprotectants (glycerol, methanol and dimethyl sulfoxide) on post-thaw quality, viability, fertilization ability and DNA damage of cryopreserved Nile tilapia (*Oreochromis niloticus*) spermatozoa. CryoLetters. 2019;**40**(1):11-17

[16] Gwo JC, Ohta H, Okuzawa K, Wu HC. Cryopreservation of sperm from the endangered formosan landlocked salmon (*Oncorhynchus masou formosanus*). Theriogenology. 1999;**51**:569-582

[17] Vivieros ATM, So N, Komen J. Sperm cryopreservation of African catfish (*Clarius gariepinus*): Cryoprotectants,

freezing rates and sperm: Egg dilution ratio. Theriogenology. 2000;**54**:1395-1408

[18] Wienholds E, Schulte-Merker S, Walderich B, Plasterk RH. Target-selected inactivation of the zebrafish rag1 gene. Science. 2002;**297**:99-102

[19] Dahm R, Geisler R. Learning from small fry: The zebrafish as a genetic model organism for aquaculture fish species. Marine Biotechnology. 2006;**8**(4):329-345

Section 2

Using of Zebrafish in Neurological Studies

Chapter 2

Alarm Test: A Novel Chemical-Free Behavioural Assessment Tool for Zebrafish

Ruchi Jakhmola-Mani, Khyati Mittal and Deepshikha Pande Katare

Abstract

Zebrafish (ZF) is an incredible animal for the study of neurological disorders. Its behaviour is like higher vertebrate animals, which makes it gainful and robust. Understanding the psychological and biological implications of housing settings for ZFs is very crucial in improving the replicability and dependability of ZF behavioural research. Individual housing triggers depression-like symptoms that suggest that housing conditions have negative effects on ZF and can result in the data discrepancy. Based on various behavioural analyses, we have evaluated that the ZFs kept in isolation and the ZFs kept in herd conditions exhibit different behavioural patterns. Interestingly, normal isolated subjects exhibit similar behavioural patterns as Alzheimer disease (AD)-induced subjects; hence, this can have serious implications on any study concerning behaviour of ZFs. Therefore, we have reported a new behavioural test named "Alarm Test", which effectively discriminates normal isolated subjects from AD subjects. Alarm Test is observed to be better than other tests used for studying fear and anxiety in ZFs as it uses the indigenous compound released by ZFs during fear and makes use of the same for analysis. This can reduce the involvement of chemicals during behavioural analysis as well as sacrifice of ZFs for collection of alarm substance.

Keywords: zebrafish, behaviour, alarm test, Alzheimer's disease, predators

1. Background

The behaviour of animal and human is metaphorically related to each other. The study of animal behaviour sheds light on understanding the complex human emotions [1]. In the quest for knowledge on human cognitive abilities and to understand the functioning of the central nervous system, animals are used as a prototype to show different behaviours when subjected to experiments on stress, chemical-induced diseases, cognitive impairment, environmental toxins, thirst, hunger and many more [2]. Zebrafishes (ZFs) are small and proved to be fruitful for many high-throughput applications (**Figure 1**).

They have the tendency to remain in groups and exhibit social behaviour which is known as shoaling [3]. Thus, ZF has been used for mimicking the social behaviour of humans. Studies have reported that the anxiety level and stress response

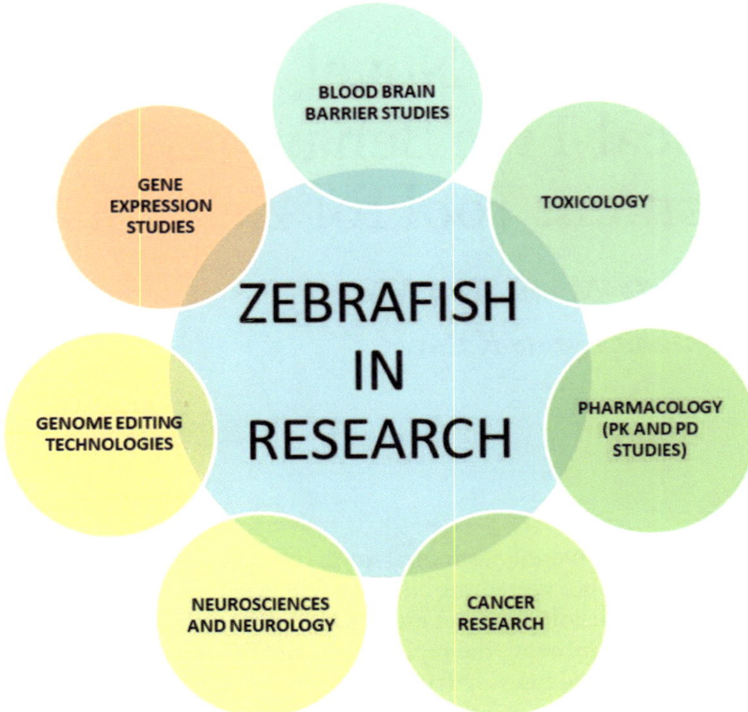
BLOOD BRAIN BARRIER STUDIES
GENE EXPRESSION STUDIES
TOXICOLOGY
ZEBRAFISH IN RESEARCH
GENOME EDITING TECHNOLOGIES
PHARMACOLOGY (PK AND PD STUDIES)
NEUROSCIENCES AND NEUROLOGY
CANCER RESEARCH

Figure 1.
Utilization of zebrafish in different sciences and domains.

can be measured in ZFs by evaluating their diving pattern in tank diving test and so forth for another test as well [4]. However, these tests have some limitations which have not been reported anywhere. For example, during our experiments we observed that control behaviour of ZF subjects when introduced in a new vessel is extensive thrashing from wall to wall of that vessel, uninterrupted and vigorous movement for around 2 minutes, heavy breathing and escape actions. This behaviour is replicated by the first few fishes introduced in the same vessel. This is regarded as an ideal control behaviour. As we add more fishes (mostly fourth, fifth and so on), this ideal control behaviour was difficult to attain. The ZFs in the same vessel were now sensing the presence of some substance presumably released by every fish that entered before them in that water, which was hindering with their ideal behaviour. We named this compound as "alarm substance". The new behaviour exhibited by them was that, as soon as the subject entered the vessel, it was abnormally silent and did not move at all for a long period of time which is mostly 3–4 minutes. Even after little encouragement, the subject moved a little and then settled at the bottom of the vessel. In this chapter, we have tried to report these limitations as well as suggestions to overcome these issues so that correct behaviour of ZFs can be studied.

Additionally, the social isolation disrupts the growth performance and innate immune response of ZFs, and it reflects in their behaviour and temporal-spatial judgements [5]. ZFs exhibit this depression in the form of increased cortisol in their body and show decreased anxiety. Stressful housing conditions, i.e. social isolation, are sometimes inevitable in experiments wherein subjects are exposed to oral doses of chemicals, a precondition in that experiment [6, 7]. Often research communities pay attention to the toxin-treated behaviour, but none has reported

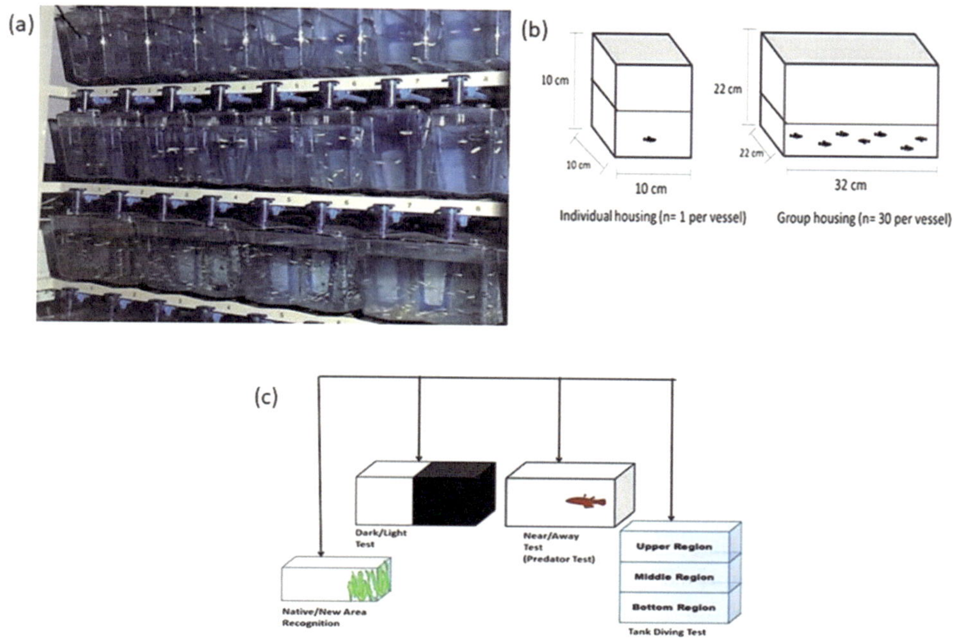

Figure 2.
(a) Zebrafish facility. (b) Zebrafishes housed individually and in group. (c) Diagrammatic representation of the behavioural test setups, i.e. native/new area, dark/light test, near/away (predator test) and tank diving test.

the differences in behaviour of control ZFs when kept in isolation and herd conditions (**Figure 2a** and **b**). The results obtained from such experiments can be misleading as the subjects already have the depression symptoms, and, therefore, through behavioural assessment of such subjects, conclusive results cannot be obtained.

The alarm substance is not very easily obtained from ZF. Typically, the scientists collect the alarm substance by inducing a stimulus of the presence of a predatory fish and then sacrificing the ZFs by creating cuts in their epidermal layers [8] or by keeping predators with ZFs [9]. Since it is not wise to keep the predator and subject in the same apparatus and also to sacrifice subjects for extraction of the alarm substance, few studies recently have also mentioned the usage of few chemicals like hypoxanthine 3-*N*-oxide which induces the similar effect [10]. This is now trending among scientific fraternity, but this also brings an issue of unforeseen effects of this compound on ZF subjects even when exposed for a short duration of time, i.e. during behavioural assessment. Therefore, in the present chapter, we have proposed a new test named *alarm test* which is chemical free and does not involve sacrificing ZF subjects for the retrieval of alarm substance and can be used for the accurate assessment of fear and anxiety in ZFs.

2. Need of behavioural assessments in animal model methods

Although rats and mice are unquestionably used as the most reliable and successful models for studying any neurodegenerative diseases, there is a need to look into some other options which are cost-effective and simple like most importantly an option to replace higher mammals as subjects in research. Zebrafish, a non-mammalian species that has already been established as vertebrate development model, opens new doors for the investigation of brain mechanisms. It is an emerging animal model for studying psychiatry and neurological behaviour. Both human and zebrafish have similarities in their psychological behaviour, because of which it becomes the most popular model for understanding the complexity of behavioural and phenotypic patterns of human brain disorders. Additionally, this species has some well-characterized features which make it cost-effective and robust. Another hope in this system is the sequence similarity of the vertebrate zebrafish with the humans.

While ZFs can be used for modelling liver cancer [11], diabetes [12, 13], cardiovascular disorders [14, 15] and other metabolic disorders [16, 17], the major contribution of this model is projected in neurodegenerative sciences. This is due to the extensive similarity of its brain structure with that of the humans [18, 19]. The incidences of neurodegenerative diseases in the growing population have increased worldwide, and it is expected that its prevalence will rise in the next few years. In different forms of neurological disorders, the most common is Alzheimer's disease which constitutes around 50–60% of the major public health issues. But still no curative treatment has been found for any of the neurodegenerative problems. For better understanding of the mechanism of action and in order to reproduce the same lesions, symptoms and causes of these pathologies, a series of animal models has been designed and used worldwide. Since the brain anatomy and behaviour of ZF and human are similar and ZFs are readily available in large numbers, therefore ZFs are favoured over other animal models. Their study can shed some light on understanding the complex human pathologies and subsequent behaviour. Since neurodegenerative diseases have a typical behavioural pattern and symptoms, therefore the ZF models are also scrutinized on the basis of their replicability at behavioural levels along with the disease pathology.

Various neurodegenerative models are established on zebrafishes through different routes, i.e. oral and intraperitoneal. Often research communities pay attention to the toxin-treated behaviour, but no one has paid attention to the regular and normal behaviour of the ZF. The present study is novel and reports for the first time the differences in the behaviour of control fishes kept in alone and herd conditions. Our study also raises a question whether these subjects' behaviour is correctly judged or not.

3. Existing zebrafish-related behavioural tests

A total of four different behavioural assessment techniques were generated in our laboratory setup (**Figure 2c**). The inference from the test is also elaborated along with the test write-up. The commonly performed behavioural tests with ZFs are as follows:

3.1 New/native area recognition

The box was made of non-toxic glass and measured 30 × 22 × 22 cm. The box was divided into two equal chambers: empty area (native area) and area with plants and stones (new area). The box was kept open from above. There were two small circular openings (diameter, 4 cm) in the separator wall between the two chambers which allowed the fish to move between the two areas. A live camera was positioned above the box, which was connected to a computer so that subjects can be observed from a distance. The test ran for 10 minutes and started after the fish was placed into the new area. Activity measures (mean time spent in both areas) were hand-coded by an experimenter blind to the experimental group.

Subjects were also observed for other unusual behavioural patterns like freezing and erratic movements [20].

3.2 Dark and light test

The box was made of non-toxic glass and measured 30 × 22 × 22 cm. The box was divided into two equal chambers: a dark chamber and a light chamber. The box was kept open from above at the light chamber. There was a small circular opening (diameter, 4 cm) in the separator wall between the two chambers which allowed the fish to move between the light and dark partitions. A live camera was positioned above the light/dark box, which was connected to a computer so that subjects can be observed from a distance. The test ran for 10 minutes and started after the fish was placed into the light chamber. After completion of the task, the fish was returned to its test facility. Activity measures (mean time spent in both chambers) in the light and dark compartments were hand-coded during the experiment by an experimenter blind to the experimental group. Subjects were also observed for other unusual behavioural patterns [10].

3.3 Tank diving test

The protocol for the novel tank diving test used was modified from Egan et al. [21]. Fishes were transferred to the test tank which measured 60 × 30 × 46 cm (length × width × height). As soon as the fish was transferred to the apparatus, the live camera was started, and subject was monitored from a distance. The camera filmed the tank from the front which was already marked for three sections: bottom, middle and upper. Subjects could freely explore the tank for 10 minutes. The test was analysed on the three parameters: time spent in the bottom area; time spent in the middle area; and time spent in the upper area of the tank. Plus, the subject's frequency of shifting in all the three sections was hand-recorded separately [22].

3.4 Predator avoidance test

The box was made of non-toxic glass and measured 30 × 22 × 22 cm. The area was filled with water. A live camera was positioned above the chamber, which was connected to a computer so that subjects can be observed from a distance. The test ran for 10 mins and started after the fish was placed into the chamber. After 2 minutes *C. punctatus* (predator) was introduced in front of the subject so close that it can sense its presence. The behavioural activity aroused after the introduction of object, and it was monitored and comprehended. Activity measures (mean time spent near the subject/away from the subject) were hand-coded during the experiment by an experimenter blind to the experimental group. Subjects were also observed for other unusual behavioural patterns [10].

4. Anomalies in behavioural assessment setups

4.1 Comparison of models and assessment of robustness of test results

For differentiating between models and behavioural tests, 8–12-month-old wild-type ZFs (n = 90) were procured from a certified vendor. All the conditions and procedures were maintained according to the Institutional Animal Ethics Committee. ZFs were acclimatized for 2–3 months in laboratory conditions. Water temperature was maintained at 28°C. ZFs ranged in weight from 0.3 to 0.5 g and were divided equally into three groups (n = 30) labelled as herd control (HC), isolated control (IC) and Alzheimer's disease (AD) model [23]. In both AD and HC group, ZFs were kept together in the same tank, while in the IC group, ZFs were kept individually in 30 small vessels. Standard conditions of 12 hours of light/dark cycles were maintained, and food was provided twice a day. The fishes were not collected as part of a faunal survey. Also, fishes were not harmed or sacrificed for the current experiment. The experimental conditions did not distress any subject to cause lasting harm. Predator fishes were not used for behavioural analysis neither any chemical was used for induction of fear. Graphs were prepared using GraphPad Prism 6, and statistical analysis was performed with student's t-tests (*$P < 0.05$, **$P < 0.01$, ***$P < 0.001$). The error bars represent the standard error mean.

There are various ZF animal model studies that require route-dependent caging. For example, subjects dosed orally in water are kept in separate vessels, and those dosed intraperitoneally are kept together in the same vessels (**Figure 2**). During our experiments, it was observed that the control ZFs which were kept alone (IC group) for more than 3 weeks had some issues in learning and retaining feeding trainings. Their memory and cognition got worse with time, and a period came when it was very difficult to judge the differences between isolated control subjects (IC group) and cognitively impaired subjects (AD group; $AlCl_3$ induced). Thereafter special attention was given to the behaviour of IC, HC and AD groups of ZFs. The subjects were assessed on nine different parameters [20]. The following parameters were observed for 3 weeks and are discussed in **Table 1**.

It was observed that subjects kept in HC group exhibited ideal normal behaviour. Their anxiety levels were very high and different from those kept in IC group for 3 weeks. Isolated control subjects from IC group displayed less erratic movement, freezing, head-butting, thrashing, etc. During the experiment subjects were also tested for few already established behavioural tests like dark/light, new/native area, predator (near/away) and tank diving test (**Figure 3**).

We observed that isolation was causing depression in socially secluded IC group. The behavioural tests like tank diving test and novel object test gave an indication

	Isolated control (IC) group			**Herd control (HC) group**			**Alzheimer's disease (AD) group**		
	Days								
Parameters	7	14	21	7	14	21	7	14	21
Anxiety	+++	++	+	+	+	+	+++	++	+
Hypo-locomotion	NA	+	++	NA	NA	NA	+	++	+++
Erratic movement	+++	++	+	NA	NA	NA	+++	++	+
Freezing	+++	+	+	NA	NA	NA	+++	++	+
Backward swimming	NA	NA	NA	NA	NA	NA	+	++	+++
Photokinesis	+++	++	+	+++	+++	+++	+++	++	+
Thrashing	+++	+	+	NA	NA	NA	+++	+	+
Adaptation to social environment	+++	++	+	NA	NA	NA	+++	++	+
Head-butting	+++	++	+	NA	NA	NA	+++	++	+

Table 1.
Analysis of ZF behaviour when put to isolation conditions (IC) and herd conditions (HC) and in Alzheimer's disease (AD) model.

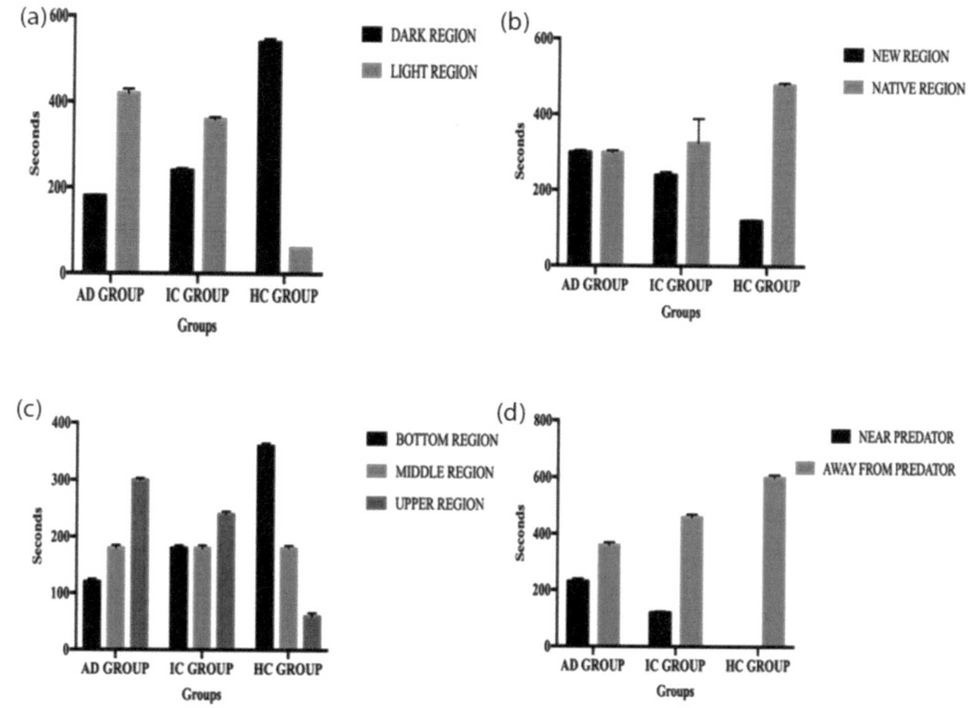

Figure 3.
Behavioural tests conducted between herd control (HC), isolated control (IC) and Alzheimer's disease (AD) model group. (a) Dark/light test, (b) native/new area test, (c) tank diving test, (d) predator avoidance test.

that the behaviour of isolated subjects was almost like the AD model ZF's. For example, the ideal behaviour of ZFs in tank diving test is to swim at the bottom, i.e. away from predator. AD model ZFs are generally found at the upper region of the tank since they do not feel fear as the disease progresses (**Figure 3c**). The similar pattern was observed for isolated subjects of IC group. Likewise, when IC and AD groups were compared using predator avoidance test, both IC and AD groups were very much alike (**Figure 3d**). Similarly, both IC and AD groups were unable to locate their native area in new/native area test (**Figure 3b**). Also, during light and dark test, there was not much difference between IC and AD group (**Figure 3a**). These findings indicate that if someone setups an experiment for assessing the behaviour of neurodegenerative and cognitively impaired ZF subjects and then if controls are also kept in isolation, then it will be difficult to categorize them based on the behavioural results, and the results obtained from such experiments will be misleading.

There was one more critical observation: i.e. usually the test setups published worldwide have a single test apparatus wherein all the fishes are tested for behavioural parameters. Typically, the water is never changed in that apparatus during an experiment. Interestingly, during behavioural assessment it was observed that fishes have a special way of communicating. Every time a new fish from HC group was added to the test apparatus (light/dark, new/native, etc.), their ideal behaviour changed dramatically. The behaviour of the first few fish in all the tests was exhibiting their ideal behaviour, i.e. extreme thrashing and anxiety, while the fishes (from same group: herd control (HC)) added later to the same test were showing different behaviour, i.e. remaining still at one location for 2–3 minutes and did not move much. Although these subjects are from cognitively alert group, i.e. HC

Group, even then, their behaviour was not close to their ideal behaviour. Therefore, an inference was made that the first few fishes released something in the water which was interfering with the behaviour of other fishes. These results prompted our study to formulate a new test for understanding this unusual behaviour.

This new test is called as "alarm test", and it was utilized to answer few issues invoked during the study. The first issue was to differentiate correctly between cognitively impaired subjects and socially isolated subjects. The second was to evaluate the presence and potency of the alarm substance, and the last was to emphasize on changing the water from behavioural setups after introduction of each fish during behavioural assessment.

5. Making of the novel "alarm test"

5.1 Collection of alarm substance

A test setup was created (**Figure 4**) for collection of test-water. It was done by adding ZFs one by one in the vessels. It was observed that the first fish to enter in the first vessel exhibited lot of anxiety-provoked thrashing and erratic swimming. But the next fish after the first one displayed lesser anxiety and was more attentive than the first one. The silence in their behaviour grew with each added subject in that vessel. It was concluded that every fish which entered the vessel was leaving some sort of signal in the water that was alarming them for any danger. The silence in their behaviour was not calmness; instead, it was the fear of a probable predator as they displayed extreme stillness and jumping movements simultaneously.

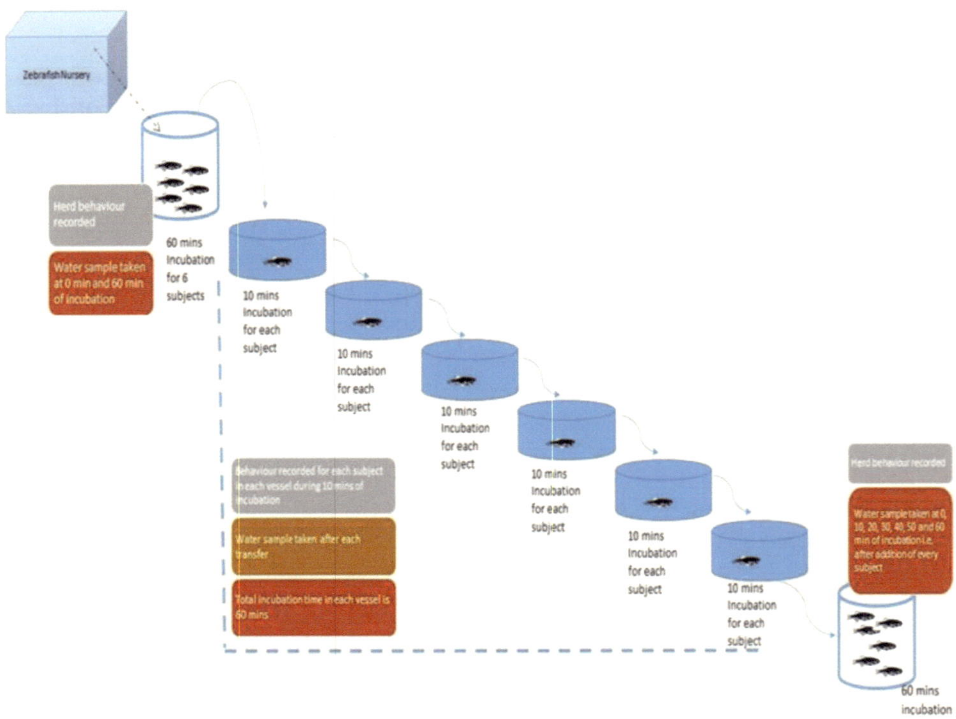

Figure 4.
Illustrative diagram on devising a protocol for collection of alarm substance in test water from ZFs.

5.2 Alarm test setup

A new test was formulated to understand how zebrafishes communicate fear and anxiety with each other. Their behaviour was extensively studied by setting-up a test protocol which comprised of two big glass vessels (water capacity: 1 litre) (14.5 × 10.5 × 14.5 cm) and six small vessels (water capacity: 100 ml) (10 × 10 × 10 cm). The vessels were kept open from above. Two big vessels were filled with 400 ml water and small vessels had 50 ml water each. Less water was kept for inducing stress to the subject (both space and new area stress) (**Figure 4**).

5.3 Alarm test protocol

The test ran for 130 minutes and started after six fishes were placed into the first big vessel one by one (**Figure 4**). The fishes were added to the first big vessel in the interval of 10 minutes each, and water sample was collected consecutively. After 60 minutes of incubation, one subject was transferred to the first small vessel and kept there for 10 minutes. Later it was taken out and transferred to the second small vessel and likewise was left in each of the six small vessels for 10 minutes each. Eventually the first subject was transferred to the last big vessel and rested there till all the ZFs reach the last big vessel. Similar steps were followed for rest of the five fishes. Every time a fish was transferred from one vessel to the other, the water sample was collected, and subjects' behaviour was documented. The water sample collected from all the vessels in short intervals of 10 minutes was later stored and was labelled as test-water. The similar protocol was repeated five times. Thereafter to examine the test-water, the new set of ZFs was taken from the nursery and was put to two different conditions. One subject was put in the first vessel with fresh water, and the other was put in the second vessel with test-water. The water in the first vessel was changed for every new fish, while the second vessel with test-water was not changed. Results were replicated with random subjects from the nursery, and it was confirmed that the test-water was able to induce fear-like symptoms in ZFs.

6. Advantage of alarm test over other tests

The alarm test was later compared to the predator avoidance test. For that we took two separate vessels. The first vessel was similar to the predator avoidance test, and the second vessel had test-water. The ZFs in the first vessel exhibited thrashing and maintained distance from the predator, but after analysing the subject for a few minutes, it became normal. However in the second vessel, the ZF subject did not show any thrashing and head-butting; instead, the subject displayed increased alertness and fear symptoms, i.e. the subject was extremely silent and was pinned at one location immediately after putting in the water. It continued for approximately 10 minutes, and after that it acclimatized in the environment. The similar test was repeated for HC, IC and AD group. It was observed that the HC group responded to both predator and alarm test very well. The IC group did not respond very well for predator test (*C. punctatus*) but was able to respond equally well for alarm test. On the contrary, the AD group did not respond to either predator (*C. punctatus*) or alarm test. Therefore, this test-water was proven to be useful in detecting cognitively impaired subjects over socially isolated subjects (**Figure 5**).

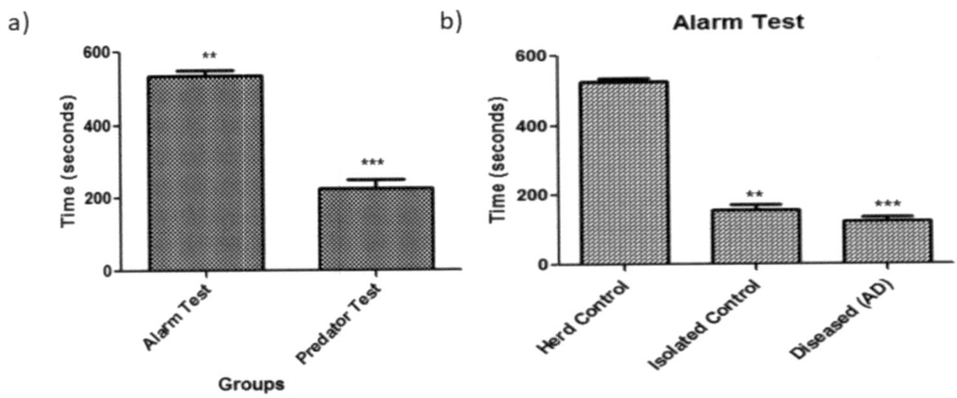

Figure 5.
(a) Comparison between alarm test and predator test. (b) Differences in sensitivity of alarm test for AD (Alzheimer's disease), IC (isolated control) and HC (herd control) models ($P < 0.01^{**}$) ($P < 0.001^{***}$).

Lastly, it is very important to note that research groups which work on ZF behavioural analysis must change the water after each testing as this might interfere with the ideal behaviour of ZF.

7. Conclusion

Behavioural study is one of the best approaches to identify the changes occurring in the body. Expanding the scope of behavioural tests is an imperative process in this area [9, 21]. In addition, ZF is presently developing as a helpful model for studying neurobehavioural changes, including typical and neurotic conditions. It shows anxiety-like behaviour, thrashing, head-butting and changes in its conducts in response to any external stimuli. Since ZF is a social animal, it is always preferred to remain in herd [24]. Our work is in accordance with this information as we are reporting behavioural changes of control ZF in herd and in isolated conditions. The isolated fishes were showing behaviour similar to ZFs from the AD model. So, it is advisable to keep them in herd while establishing any pathological model, as isolation can severely induce depression even to normal fishes used as controls which can give faulty results. Since many at times it is not feasible with every experiment to keep ZFs in herd, we have devised a new test to be called as alarm rest for behavioural analysis. It is a chemical-free test for analysing the ideal behaviour of ZFs. This test was equally effective for the fishes kept in either isolated or in herd conditions.

There are studies which suggest that fishes have the tendency to release cortisol and chondroitin sulphate in stress conditions [5]. One study has reported that chondroitin triggers fear behaviour in ZFs [25]. This substance released by one fish acts as an alarming sign for the rest against any danger. Similarly, another study by Ramsay et al. [26] had used cortisol as a parameter to evaluate the stress response in ZF [27, 28]. They reported that crowded conditions help in optimizing the health, growth and reproduction abilities of ZF. This is optimum for their overall growth. Keeping ZFs in herd conditions is a good thing, but when it comes to behavioural test, the fishes are assessed individually for all parameters. In the present work, we have observed that the substance released by the first few fishes in any behavioural test tanks interferes and alters the behaviour of the next fishes in the row. Therefore, it is advisable to keep changing the water in the vessels during tests (native/new, predator avoidance, etc.) in an experiment. This observation is novel and an intimate scientific fraternity about the limitations and errors during the behavioural assessment of animal models.

Acknowledgement

We would like to acknowledge Dr. Ashok K. Chauhan, Founder President, Amity University, Noida, Uttar Pradesh, for providing the infrastructure.

Author details

Ruchi Jakhmola-Mani, Khyati Mittal and Deepshikha Pande Katare*
Proteomics and Translational Research Lab, Amity Institute of Biotechnology, Amity University, Noida, Uttar Pradesh, India

*Address all correspondence to: dpkatare@amity.edu

References

[1] Brown RC, Lockwood AH, Sonawane BR. Neurodegenerative diseases: An overview of environmental risk factors. Environmental Health Perspectives. 2005;**113**:1250-1256

[2] Levin ED, Cerutti DT. Chapter 15. Behavioural neuroscience of zebrafish. In: Methods of Behaviour Analysis in Neuroscience. 2nd ed. CRC Press, Taylor & Francis; 2009:293

[3] Gerlai R. Zebrafish, a potential novel research tool for the analysis and modeling of anxiety. In: Different Views of Anxiety Disorders. IntechOpen; 12 Sep 2011. p. 137

[4] Blaser RE, Rosemberg DB. Measures of anxiety in zebrafish (*Danio rerio*): Dissociation of black/white preference and novel tank test. PLoS One. 2012;**17**:36931

[5] Shams S, Seguin D, Facciol A, Chatterjee D, Gerlai R. Effect of social isolation on anxiety-related behaviours, cortisol, and monoamines in adult zebrafish. Behavioural Neuroscience. 2017;**131**:49-51

[6] Clark KJ, Boczek NJ, Ekker SC. Stressing zebrafish for behavioural genetics. Reviews in the Neurosciences. 2011;**22**:49-62

[7] Hamilton TJ, Morrill A, Lucas K, Gallup J, Harris M, Healey M, et al. Establishing zebrafish as a model to study the anxiolytic effects of scopolamine. Scientific Reports. 2017;**8**:15081

[8] Speedie N, Gerlai R. Alarm substance induced behavioural responses in zebrafish (*Danio rerio*). Behavioural Brain Research. 2009;**188**:168-177

[9] Bencan Z, Sledge D, Levin ED. Buspirone, chlordiazepoxide and diazepam effects in a ZF model of anxiety. Pharmacology Biochemistry and Behavior. 2009;**94**:75-80

[10] Perra KV, Gerlai R, Adrian JC Jr. The synthetic substance hypoxanthine 3-N-oxide elicits alarm reactions in zebrafish (*Danio rerio*). Behavioural Brain Research. 2009;**205**:336-341

[11] Lu JW, Ho YJ, Yang YJ, Liao HA, Ciou SC, Lin LI, et al. Zebrafish as a disease model for studying human hepatocellular carcinoma. World Journal of Gastroenterology. 2015;**21**(42):12042

[12] Zang L, Shimada Y, Nishimura N. Development of a novel zebrafish model for type 2 diabetes mellitus. Scientific Reports. 2017;**7**(1):1461

[13] Zang L, Maddison LA, Chen W. Zebrafish as a model for obesity and diabetes. Frontiers in Cell and Developmental Biology. 20 Aug 2018;**6**:91

[14] Bournele D, Beis D. Zebrafish models of cardiovascular disease. Heart Failure Reviews. 2016;**21**(6):803-813

[15] Salman HE, Yalcin HC. Advanced blood flow assessment in zebrafish via experimental digital particle image velocimetry and computational fluid dynamics modeling. Micron. 2019:102801

[16] Williams MB, Watts SA. Current basis and future directions of zebrafish nutrigenomics. Genes & Nutrition. 2019;**14**(1):34

[17] Wang C, Zhao Y, Jin Y. The emerging PFOS alternative OBS exposure induced gut microbiota dysbiosis and hepatic metabolism disorder in adult zebrafish. Comparative Biochemistry and Physiology Part C: Toxicology & Pharmacology. 2020;**230**:108703

[18] Ahi EP, Brunel M, Tsakoumis E, Schmitz M. Transcriptional study of appetite regulating genes in the brain of zebrafish (*Danio rerio*) with impaired leptin signalling. Scientific Reports. 2019;**9**(1):1-14

[19] Mazzolini J, Le Clerc S, Morisse G, Coulonges C, Kuil LE, van Ham TJ, et al. Gene expression profiling reveals a conserved microglia signature in larval zebrafish. Glia. 2020;**68**(2):298-315

[20] Spence R, Gerlach G, Lawrence C, Smith C. The behaviour and ecology of the zebrafish, *Danio rerio*. Biological Reviews. 2008;**83**:13-34

[21] Egan RJ, Bergner CL, Hart PC, Cachat JM, Canavello PR, Elegante MF. Understanding behavioural and physiological phenotypes of stress and anxiety in zebrafish. Behavioural Brain Research. 2009;**205**:38-44

[22] Blank M, Guerim LD, Cordeiro RF, Vianna MR. A one-trial inhibitory avoidance task to zebrafish: Rapid acquisition of an NMDA-dependent long-term memory. Neurobiology of Learning and Memory. 2009;**92**:529-534

[23] Jakhmola-Mani R, Mittal K, Katare DP. Protective effects of quercetin in zebrafish model of Alzheimer's disease. Asian Journal of Pharmaceutics. 2018;**12**:661-666

[24] Kalueff AV, Gebhardt M, Stewart AM, Cachat JM, Brimmer M, Chawla JS, et al. Towards a comprehensive catalog of zebrafish behaviour 1.0 and beyond. Zebrafish. 2013;**10**:70-86

[25] Mathuru AS, Kibat C, Cheong WF, Shui G, Wenk MR, Friedrich RW, et al. Chondroitin fragments are odorants that trigger fear behaviour in fish. Current Biology. 2012;**22**(6):538-544

[26] Ramsay JM, Feist GW, Varga ZM, Westerfield M, Kent ML, Schreck CB. Whole-body cortisol is an indicator of crowding stress in adult zebrafish, *Danio rerio*. Aquaculture. 2006;**258**:565-574

[27] Kalueff AV, Wheaton M, Murphy DL. What's wrong with my mouse model? Advances and strategies in animal modeling of anxiety and depression. Behavioural Brain Research. 2007;**179**:1-18

[28] Kalueff AV, Schmidt MV. Novel experimental models and paradigms for neuropsychiatric disorders: Editorial. Progress in Neuropsychopharmacology and Biological Psychiatry. 2011;**35**:1355-1356

Section 3

Using of Zebrafish in Miscellaneous Diseases

Chapter 3

The Zebrafish Kupffer's Vesicle: A Special Organ in a Model Organism to Study Human Diseases

Mónica Roxo-Rosa and Susana Santos Lopes

Abstract

The Kupffer's vesicle (KV) is a small, ciliated organ transiently present during embryogenesis of the zebrafish and other teleosts. The KV is required to the establishment of visceral laterality, such as the heart on the left side, being also known by the name left-right organizer (LRO). The LRO is found in other vertebrates, including mice, rabbits, frogs and human embryos. Among these, the KV became an excellent model organ to investigate the early left-right events during development and in disease. Many ciliary molecular players associated to the human disease primary ciliary dyskinesia have been tested in the zebrafish looking at KV cilia and its downstream effects on flow and left-right markers. Additionally, given its morphology and molecular features, we proposed the KV as a model organ to study the molecular mechanisms of the renal cyst inflation that occurs in the autosomal dominant polycystic kidney disease. Although having no connection to the kidney, the KV mimics a renal cyst because it is a fluid-filled vesicle, lined by monociliated epithelial cells that express polycystin-2, which knockdown leads to the organ luminal enlargement through changes in ion/water epithelial transport. Here, we explore the usefulness of the zebrafish KV to model these diseases.

Keywords: Kupffer's vesicle (KV), left-right (LR), left-right organizer (LRO), primary ciliary dyskinesia (PCD), autosomal dominant polycystic kidney disease (ADPKD)

1. The Kupffer's vesicle

The KV is an organ transiently present in the early embryonic life of the fish to establish internal body laterality [1, 2]. It derives from the dorsal forerunner cells (DFCs), a cluster of cells that migrate together from shield developmental stage until the end of the epiboly stage during zebrafish development. The DFC cluster later forms a lumen, and cilia start to protrude from the cells apically towards the new space. Thus, the KV organ will be formed by only one cell layer surrounding a lumen (**Figure 1**). The lumen is also progressively filled with fluid as it opens up through a mechanism involving cystic fibrosis transmembrane conductance regulator (CFTR, OMIM-602421), as described before [3–5]. CFTR is a chloride channel

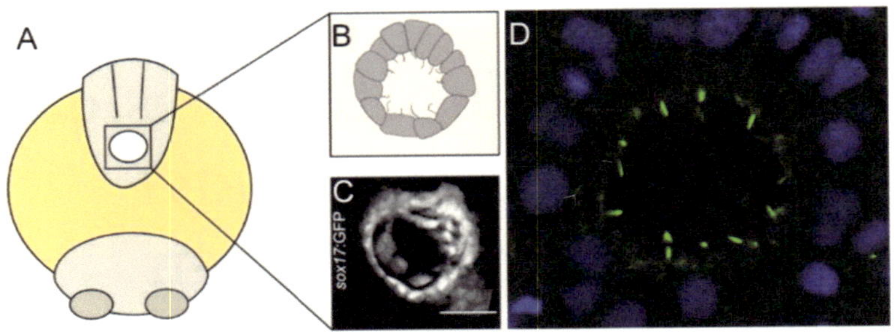

Figure 1.
The zebrafish Kupffer's vesicle. (A) It is imaged from the dorsal side of the embryo in the tail region from 6 to 14 hours post fertilization (hpf). (B) KV is formed by one layer of monociliated cells. (C) In sox17:GFP transgenic line, KV-lining cells are labeled with GFP. (D) Cross section through the KV midplane acquired by confocal fluorescent microscopy shows the cilia stained with acetylated alpha-tubulin in green and nuclei stained with DAPI in blue.

which absence or dysfunction causes cystic fibrosis [6–8]. As the KV enlarges, the solitary cilium from each KV cell starts to beat, and by ten somite stage (ss), there are on average 80% motile cilia and 20% immotile cilia in a total of 60 cells [9]. Despite it presents different shapes and sizes, the left-right organizer (LRO) has a conserved function among vertebrates, which is to break initial symmetry of embryonic body plans. As detailed below there are still many gaps in the developmental process of left-right (LR) establishment that need to be tested. Due to its genetic amenability and optical transparency, the zebrafish has gained impact in the LR field as one of the best models for testing early LR establishment questions [2, 9–15]. So far, it is the only animal system where we can manipulate the LRO without damaging or sacrificing the animal, thus letting it develop until organ localization can be visualized [2]. This allows for causal conclusions to be drawn in the same individual fish, which is a powerful advantage in developmental biology.

2. Primary cilia dyskinesia

2.1 The disease

Primary ciliary dyskinesia (PCD) is a rare congenital and heterogeneous disorder (OMIM: 244400) with an estimated prevalence of around 1:10,000 according to Rubbo and Lucas [16], which is thought to be higher in consanguineous populations [17]. However, other references in the literature consider a much lower prevalence, affecting approximately 1 in 20,000 individuals [18]. It is thought that the correct prevalence of the disease is unknown because many patients remain undiagnosed. PCD is characterized by a deficient mucociliary clearance, which is caused by the lack of motile cilia in the respiratory epithelia, uncoordinated ciliary pattern, or a total lack of ciliary motion giving rise to static cilia. PCD leads to chronic respiratory infections, and the earlier it is diagnosed, the better prognostic the patients will have. Its clinical features usually begin at birth with respiratory distress followed by a wet cough in early childhood and evolve to include bronchiectasis and chronic sinusitis. In the worst scenario, PCD may lead to lung lobectomy [19].

However, PCD is not just a respiratory disease because half of the PCD cases are associated with situs inversus and heterotaxy, and in these latter cases, there is a high correlation with congenital heart disease [16]. Male sterility is common in adults because normal sperm flagella are special motile cilia and in PCD patients may present defective motility. Female ectopic pregnancies have also been reported due to the presence of defective motile cilia lining the fallopian tubes [20]. PCD usually follows an autosomal recessive inheritance pattern [17].

To date, mutations in more than 35 genes were identified to cause PCD. These genes are mainly coding for axonemal proteins that are required for cilia motility or for proteins that are needed for the assembly or transport of axonemal components [18, 21–23].

Our body is LR asymmetrical. In humans, the heart, spleen, and pancreas are localized on the left, while most of the liver and gallbladder are placed on the right side of our body axis. The fact that patients with immotile cilia presented defects in the location of their internal organs was not obvious to discern and raised many questions in the 1970s.

Bjorn Afzelius, who devoted great interest to this topic, postulated that the existence of an embryonic organ covered by motile ciliated epithelia should explain the laterality defects seen in patients with the immotile cilia syndrome [24]. However, until today the complete molecular mechanism is still to be fully demonstrated.

2.2 The KV as a model organ to study PCD

Previous early experiments on animal models, namely, in mice mutants named *inversus viscerum*, have shown that mutants that have no ciliary motility in the primitive node showed defective situs [25]. Imaging of the mouse nodal cilia helped to establish this causal link. These were first imaged in fixed samples by performing in situ hybridization with a riboprobe for LR-dynein (*lrd*) [25]. Soon after, mice nodal cilia and nodal flow were filmed and observed in live embryos for the first time by Nonaka et al. [26]. These authors compared wild-type (WT) embryos with homozygous mutants for KIF3b that formed no cilia and had no nodal flow. However, a definitive evidence that the nodal flow was relevant came from the elegant experiment, where Nonaka et al. [27] reversed the fluid flow that was generated by the nodal motile cilia using an artificial flow in immotile mutants. This study revealed that the correct direction of the fluid flow was crucial for the correct establishment of LR. Since then many mouse mutants were generated and studied [28, 29]. Research on other model organisms, such as frogs and zebrafish, followed in order to pursue the molecular mechanisms of laterality (e.g., [2, 30]). Among all the models in place, the zebrafish and its KV offer unique advantages to the LR field that we will explain and focus here.

The KV is ventrally positioned deep in the embryo, close to the yolk (**Figure 1**), but nevertheless it is accessible for live imaging from the dorsal side. This is only possible due to its optical clarity. The embryo is extremely transparent allowing filming the cilia inside the KV in a live intact zebrafish embryo that is simply mounted in soft agarose and embryo medium. This is strikingly different from any other vertebrate model. Mice require extracting the embryos at 7.5 days after coitus from the mother's uterus, and then dissected embryos are mounted in a medium prior to removal of the Reichert's membrane that covers the node, to then allow to film the cilia that lay inside the node [26]. In *Xenopus*, it is needed to dissect a frog embryo at stage 14 and perform dorsal explant cultures [30]. Therefore, in both these model organisms, the manipulations needed to expose the node for live imaging will later lead to the death of the animal, before the organs are placed in their asymmetric destinations. This problem impedes causal conclusions in the same individuals.

Zebrafish KV, due to its optical properties for live imaging, has been extremely useful for the study of nodal flow dynamics (**Figure 2**). How flow forces could trigger the first signals in the KV cells has been intensively explored in this model by our lab, both using experimental and theoretical approaches [2, 31–33].

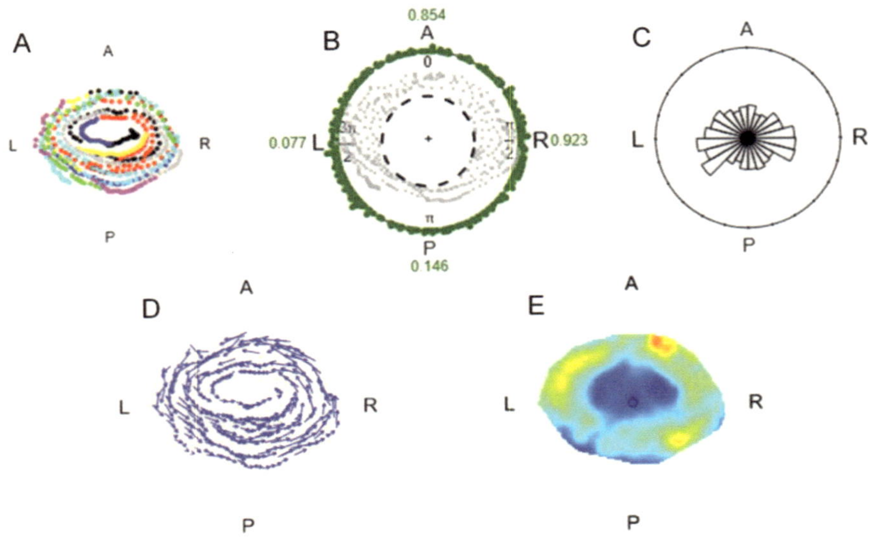

Figure 2.
Experimental fluid flow measurements and their different readouts. (A) Native particle tracking where each second has a different color to rapidly show where are the slowest regions of flow in the KV. (B) Rayleigh tests were performed considering a null hypothesis of a bias distribution toward a given KV quadrant, and p values are indicated as green numbers. Note that only particles moving at a distance of r > 0.5 from the center of the KVs were considered (r is the normalized distance from the center (r = 0) to the wall (r = 1) of the KV). (C) Rose maps show where flow is stronger in a radial manner. (D) Vector maps denote the actual flow forces in a vectorial manner. (E) Heat maps of flow speed showing detailed regions within each KV. The pseudocolor scale represents flow speed in micrometers per *second, where red represents high speed* versus *low speed in blue. A, anterior; P, posterior; R, right; L, left.*

We focused this review on the LR studies that deal with early events that occur in the KV organ. The nature of the signal that is perceived by the KV/node cells is not yet resolved. It can still be mechanical or chemical (or both) as debated for many years, since the first mouse studies [25, 26, 34]. It is now consensual that fluid flow is important, either by its force or by transporting molecules or molecules inside extracellular vesicles [34–36].

Zebrafish studies on the speed of flow *per* KV regions have shown that flow has a stereotyped pattern that is biologically relevant for LR establishment [2]. When we stopped motility of cilia everywhere except in the right half of the KV, we could demonstrate that this led to larva with situs inversus [9]. Although this seems to advocate for a mechanosensation process, it is still possible that some chemical component exists. For example, secretion of molecules caused by shear stress triggered by the local ciliary beating. This hypothesis is currently under investigation in our lab, and it was put forward in a theoretical recent study led by our collaborator mathematicians. In this study we predicted the shear stress to be greater on the anterior-dorsal side of the KV, mainly caused by the presence of a dorsal cluster of cilia [32].

The KV system has also been used to demonstrate that cilia length impacts greatly on fluid flow speed [31, 37, 38]. Other labs have also contributed to these biophysical characterizations, such as the Amack lab by analyzing the cell shape changes that lead to the dorsal cluster of cilia [13], reported earlier by Kreiling et al. [39]. The Vermot lab by pioneering the studies on KV flow [40] and recently by studying cilia tilt along the 3D KV [12] and its resultant theoretical flow forces. Contradictory interpretations emerged from our lab [9] and Vermot lab [12] concerning the number of immotile cilia in the KV and the consequent ability for the animal to sense flow in a mechanosensory way. This subject needs further experiments to be solved as our labs used different imaging protocols to determine the number of immotile cilia. Another important contribution trying to understand the immediate output of the flow came from the Sun and Bruckner labs, where Yuan et al. have reported asymmetric intracellular calcium transients that seem to be stronger on the left side and become absent upon *pkd2* knockdown (the gene encoding polycystin 2) [41].

In summary, studies in the KV allowed for the biophysical characterization of fluid flow and have shown that disruption of these properties always lead to defective gene expression of *dand5*, the first asymmetric gene to appear in zebrafish [35]. The expression of *dand5* is thought to be dependent on flow forces and will directly impact on *nodal/spaw* later expressed in the lateral plate mesoderm. However, the nature of the crucial signal that initiates this conserved genetic cascade is still to be demonstrated.

3. Autosomal dominant polycystic kidney disease

3.1 The disease

Autosomal dominant polycystic kidney disease (ADPKD) has been reported to affect 1 in 400–1000 newborns worldwide. However, a recent population-based study in European Union puts ADPKD in the group of rare diseases, having an estimated prevalence rate of less than 1 in 2000 individuals [42]. In any case, ADPKD is for sure the most common genetic cause of renal failure [42], representing a major health problem, with an important socioeconomic impact worldwide.

It is caused by mutations in the human genes *PKD1* (OMIM-601313) and *PKD2* (OMIM-613095). These encode two ciliary proteins, polycystin-1 and polycystin-2, respectively. *PKD1* mutations account for about 78% of ADPKD patients and are associated with more severe phenotypes. In contrast, a milder disease is observed in the patients presenting PKD2 mutations (about 15% of ADPKD patients) [43]. In 2016, *GANAB* (OMIM-104160) was identified as a third gene that, when mutated, causes ADPKD [44]. This encodes the catalytic α subunit of glucosidase II, a resident enzyme of the endoplasmic reticulum involved in the *N*-glycosylation of membrane proteins [44]. Together, PKD1 and PKD2 form a ciliary mechanosensor-calcium channel complex in the renal epithelium that is essential for the intracellular calcium homeostasis [45, 46]. On the other hand, the glucosidase II subunit α is critical for the proper maturation and ciliary *versus* cell membrane localization of both PKD1 and PKD2 proteins [44]. Through not fully understood mechanisms, the absence of functional ciliary PKD1/PKD2 complex triggers the formation and inexorable expansion of multiple cysts in all segments of the nephrons [45, 46]. This ciliopathy also affects other organs and systems. The extrarenal manifestations of ADPKD include liver and pancreatic cysts, hypertension, vascular problems, and abdominal hernias [43].

The kidney cyst inflation with water and ions and continuous expansion throughout the patient life is assured by an abnormal transepithelial fluid secretion toward their lumen [47]. CFTR plays a central role in the ADPKD cyst inflation [48–53]. Early in the cystogenesis process, CFTR becomes abnormally activated in ADPKD cyst-lining cells [48–53]. Supporting the involvement of CFTR in ADPKD cyst inflation, it was shown that the fluid accumulation within cysts involves CFTR-like chloride currents [53] and it is slowed down either through inhibition or knockdown of CFTR [49–53]. Additionally, a milder renal phenotype was observed in patients affected by both ADPKD and cystic fibrosis [47].

The in vivo mechanisms involved in the abnormal activation of CFTR during kidney cyst inflation are still emerging. It is known that the lack of calcium homeostasis raises the intracellular levels of cAMP in ADPKD cells [47]. As CFTR activation requires its prior cAMP-dependent phosphorylation by PKA [5, 7, 54, 55], it has been suggested that CFTR is a downstream effector of the raised levels of cAMP, in cyst growth [47]. This led to several studies testing drugs targeting renal cAMP production. However, so far only one drug showed an effect in slowing down the enlargement of cysts in adult ADPKD patients, the Tolvaptan [56]. Acting as a vasopressin V2 receptor antagonist, Tolvaptan lowers the intracellular cAMP levels of the cyst-lining cells and, therefore, the CFTR activity [47].

An evidence is growing that renal cyst formation starts in utero and that hypertension in childhood correlated well with disease severity. This is changing the old paradigm that considers ADPKD has a late-onset disease [57]. However, renal cysts still become clinically detectable only in adulthood, when the disease is fully established. The renal volume determination by imaging techniques (ultrasound, CT, and T2-weighted NMR scans) is the available tool to assess the disease progression. Although the majority of patients remain a- or pauci-symptomatic until adulthood, the natural progression of the disease leads to the total destruction of the renal parenchyma by the countless large cysts. Ultimately, about 50% of patients end up requiring renal replacement therapy in their sixth decade of life. The recent approval of Tolvaptan in Japan, Canada, and European Union brought some hope to patients [48]. However, it shows a moderate effect in slowing down the cyst enlargement [56]. Moreover, its side effects include polydipsia, polyuria, nocturia, pollakiuria [56], and significant liver enzyme elevation [58] limiting the eligible patients to those having <50 years, CKD stages 1–3, and rapidly progressing disease [43]. This means that the identification of biomarkers for the early events of ADPKD is an unmet need of the field. These are needed for the early diagnosis of the disease and accurate prediction of renal function decline and may bring novel therapeutic targets for ADPKD.

There is, therefore, an urgent need to investigate the cellular and biochemical pathways involved in kidney cytogenesis with innovative conceptual and methodological approaches. In this review, we will put forward the zebrafish model and its KV as an unconventional but promising organ model to find such biomarkers.

3.2 The zebrafish *pkd* genes

The zebrafish genome presents seven *pkd* and *pkd-like* genes: *pkd1* (also known as *pkd1a*), *pkd1b*, *pkd1l1*, *pkd1l2a*, *pkd1l2b*, *pkd2*, and *pkd2l1* [59]. In situ hybridizations showed that both *pkd1* and *pkd2* are expressed in the zebrafish pronephros at 24 hpf. In contrast, none of the other five *pkd* genes were found to be expressed in the developing pronephros [59].

The combined knockdown of the paralogues *pkd1a* and *pkd1b*, *i.e.*, the orthologues of human *PKD1*, by injection of specific morpholinos against their mRNA which specifically block their translation, resulted in dorsal axis curved embryos [60]. An identical phenotype was observed by us and others in *pkd2* knocked-down embryos (*pkd2*-morphants) (**Figure 3**) [1, 11, 61, 62]. This phenotype was shown to be associated with changes in extracellular matrix upon the loss of these polycystins and may correlate to the vascular problems observed in ADPKD patients [60]. It ended up to being a good control of the efficiency of the knockdown of those genes in the embryo.

Additionally, the knockdown of *pkd2* leads to the formation of pronephric dilations which clearly impaired the fluid homeostasis of the animals. Indeed, *pkd2* morphants presented severe edema [11, 61, 62]. However, those pronephric dilations did not form individualized cystic structures that bud off from the tubules. Although

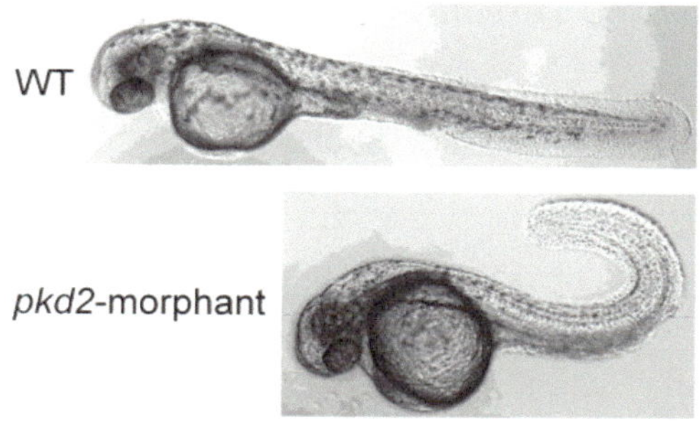

Figure 3.
Curly-up tail curvature characteristic of pkd2 morphants. Lateral view of WT and pkd2-morphant zebrafish embryos at 48 hpf.

many times named as kidney cysts, these pronephric dilations do not recapitulate the vesicular architecture of the ADPKD cysts [11, 61, 62]. On the other hand, the available zebrafish *pkd2* mutant, the curly-up ($cup^{-/-}$) mutant, did not develop kidney cysts or dilations [11, 62]. Our data suggested that this could be a result of the maternal contribution of *pkd2* mRNA present during early embryonic stages of $cup^{-/-}$ mutants [1]. The combined knockdown of *pkd1a* and *pkd1b* also resulted in the formation of kidney cysts, but, in this case, the phenotype was observed in only 10–20% of the embryos [60]. Therefore, we consider the zebrafish pronephros limited to the study of the molecular mechanisms involved in the ADPKD cystogenesis.

Although KV does not express *pkd1a*, *pkd1b*, *pkd1l2a*, *pkd1l2b*, or *pkd2l1*, by in situ hybridizations, it was shown that KV cells do express both *pkd2* [1, 59] and *pkd1l1* [59]. Clearly showing the important role of Pkd2 in the LR axis establishment, *pkd2* morphant presented laterality defects [1, 11, 62, 63]. Indeed, we showed that 33 and 21% of these embryos have right-sided and central hearts, respectively [1]. Schottenfeld and co-authors demonstrated that the laterality defects of *pkd2* morphants were comparable to those observed in $cup^{-/-}$ mutants [11]. Supporting its role in the laterality axis establishment, we detected Pkd2 protein expression through the KV-lining cells, intracellularly and along their cilia [1]. We now show in **Figure 4** that these cells do also express Pkd1l1 (polycystin 1 like 1) along their cilia. A similar expression pattern was described by Kamura et al. for this gene in the KV of medaka fish [64]. These data suggests that the Pkd1l1 is the partner of Pkd2 in the zebrafish KV cells [59], as it was also proposed for the medaka KV [64]. Supporting this hypothesis, the lack of *pkd1l1* expression caused laterality defects in medaka embryos [64].

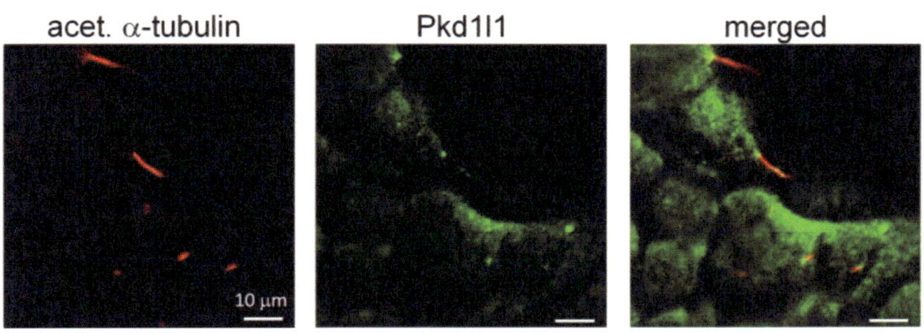

Figure 4.
Confocal images for the immunolocalization of Pkd1l1 in KV cells at the 10–11 ss in WT embryos. Pkd1l1 is detected throughout the cells' cytoplasm and along their cilia. Pkd1l1 is in green and acetylated α-tubulin in red. Scale bars: 10 μm.

3.3 The KV as a model organ to study the ADPKD cyst inflation

In our perspective, a good model to study the in vivo molecular mechanisms involved in the ADPKD cysts inflation should:

1. Be a fluid-filled vesicle.

2. Be lined by ciliated cells that must express Pkd2/Pkd1 and CFTR.

3. Exhibit a physiological fluid flow induced Ca^{2+}-signaling mediated by Pkd2.

4. Depend on CFTR activity for its lumen inflation.

5. Allow the easy knockdown of Pkd2/Pkd1 and CFTR.

6. Allow the easy access to the organ luminal volume.

7. Above all, the knockdown of PKD1/PKD2 must increase the CFTR-mediated fluid secretion into the lumen, mimicking the ADPKD cyst inflation process.

The KV is neither related to the kidney nor to the renal function. However, as it fulfills the mentioned requirements, a few years ago we proposed the zebrafish KV as a bona fide model organ of the cyst inflation process [1].

As already mentioned, this fluid-filled vesicle organ is lined by monociliated cells [1, 2, 9]. The KV cilia are motile and generate a fluid flow that is essential for the organ function [2, 9]. These are different from the primary cilia of the nephron epithelium or the cilia present in the luminal surface of *pkd2*$^{WS25/-}$ mice ADPKD cysts [65]. Nevertheless, as primary cilia of the nephron segments, the KV cilia do express Pkd2 [1]. Interestingly, this channel is crucial for the asymmetric intracellular calcium transients that occur in the KV cells [41]. Opposing to the renal primary cilia, KV cilia are not expected to express Pkd1 [59]. However, as demonstrated in **Figure 4**, they express Pkd1l1 which is thought to be the Pkd2 partner in this organ [59, 64]. We expect Pkd1l1 knockdown to cause an abnormal LR patterning, similarly to phenotype observed in *pkd1l1*-medaka morphants [64]. By using a morpholino against CFTR, we were able to corroborate the findings of Navis et al. [4] showing that the knockdown of CFTR fully impairs the proper KV inflation [1].

The transparency of zebrafish embryos makes the KV of transgenic lines presenting GFP staining in KV-lining cells accessible by confocal live microscopy [1]. These include *ras*:GFP [1, 66], *foxji1*:GFP [1, 67], *sox17*:GFP (**Figure 5**) [68], or *TgBAC(cftr-GFP)pd1041* [4] transgenic embryos. In this way, the KV allows the measurement of its whole volume as a live readout of CFTR activity, with smaller volumes, meaning reduced CFTR activity [1].

The most important feature of the model is the fact that on average the knockdown of PKD2 leads to ~1.6 times larger KV volumes than the CFTR activation. Using a pharmacological approach, we showed that the *pkd2* morphants' KV enlargement is assured by a CFTR-mediated fluid secretion into the KV lumen, mimicking the ADPKD cyst inflation process [1].

This model was an important innovation in testing drugs that may modulate the CFTR-dependent KV inflation. We will publish soon our results with Tolvaptan among other drugs. These may give us clues on new drugs that may prevent ADPKD cyst enlargement.

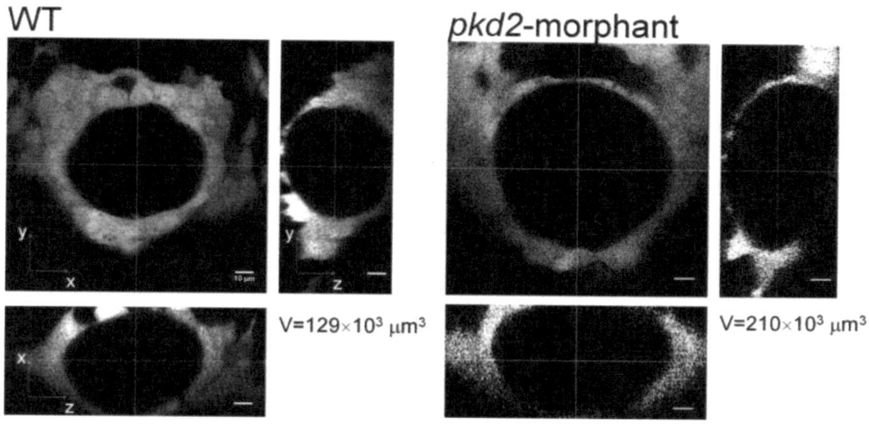

Figure 5.
KV volume. Confocal live-microscopy scans of the whole KV of 10–11 ss sox17:GFP transgenic embryos. The middle focal plane along the xy axis and the respective orthogonal views (along xz and yz axes) are shown for WT and pkd2-morphant representative embryos.

4. Conclusions

The zebrafish KV offers unique features that allow the proper study of the in vivo molecular mechanisms of both PCD and ADPKD. In the first disease, the KV has already emerged as an ideal system for its uniqueness in allowing to manipulate early genes and physical properties and then following up the LR pattern of the final organs. In the latter disease, it offers an excellent in vivo model for screening compounds and genes that may slow down cyst enlargement through CFTR inhibition.

Acknowledgements

The work was fully supported by Sociedade Portuguesa de Nefrologia (research grant 2015), iNOVA4Health - UID/Multi/04462/2013 (a program financially supported by Fundação para a Ciência e Tecnologia/Ministério da Educação e Ciência, through national funds and co-funded by FEDER under the PT2020 Partnership Agreement) and Fundação para a Ciência e Tecnologia (research grant - PTDC/BEX-BID/1411/2014). MRR was supported by national funds through Fundação para a Ciência e Tecnologia, in the context of the celebration of the program contract foreseen in the numbers 4, 5 and 6 of article 23.º of D.L. no. 57/2016 of 29 August, as amended by Law no. 57/2017 of 19 July. Zebrafish used as animal model were reared and maintained in the CEDOC Fish Facility, with the support from the research consortia Congento, co-financed by Lisboa Regional Operational Programme (Lisboa2020), under the Portugal 2020 Partnership Agreement, through the European Regional Development Fund (ERDF) and Fundação para a Ciência e Tecnologia under the project LISBOA-01-0145-FEDER-022170.

Conflict of interest

The authors declare no conflict of interest.

Author details

Mónica Roxo-Rosa* and Susana Santos Lopes*
CEDOC, Chronic Diseases Research Center, NOVA Medical School, Faculdade de Ciências Médicas, Universidade Nova de Lisboa, Lisboa, Portugal

*Address all correspondence to: monica.rosa@nms.unl.pt
and susana.lopes@nms.unl.pt

References

[1] Roxo-Rosa M, Jacinto R, Sampaio P, Lopes SS. The zebrafish Kupffer's vesicle as a model system for the molecular mechanisms by which the lack of polycystin-2 leads to stimulation of CFTR. Biology Open. 2015;**4**(11):1356-1366

[2] Sampaio P, Ferreira RR, Guerrero A, Pintado P, Tavares B, Amaro J, et al. Left-right organizer flow dynamics: How much cilia activity reliably yields laterality? Developmental Cell. 2014;**29**(6):716-728

[3] Oteíza P, Köppen M, Concha ML, Heisenberg CP. Origin and shaping of the laterality organ in zebrafish. Development. 2008;**135**(16):2807-2813

[4] Navis A, Marjoram L, Bagnat M. CFTR controls lumen expansion and function of Kupffer's vesicle in zebrafish. Development. 2013;**140**(8):1703-1712

[5] Amaral MD, Farinha CM. Rescuing mutant CFTR: A multi-task approach to a better outcome in treating cystic fibrosis. Current Pharmaceutical Design. 2013;**19**(19):3497-3508

[6] Clancy JP, Cotton CU, Donaldson SH, Solomon GM, VanDevanter DR, Boyle MP, et al. CFTR modulator theratyping: Current status, gaps and future directions. Journal of Cystic Fibrosis. 2019;**18**(1):22-34

[7] Farinha CM, King-Underwood J, Sousa M, Correia AR, Henriques BJ, Roxo-Rosa M, et al. Revertants, low temperature, and correctors reveal the mechanism of F508del-CFTR rescue by VX-809 and suggest multiple agents for full correction. Chemistry & Biology. 2013;**20**(7):943-955

[8] Roxo-Rosa M, Xu Z, Schmidt A, Neto M, Cai Z, Soares CM, et al. Revertant mutants G550E and 4RK rescue cystic fibrosis mutants in the first nucleotide-binding domain of CFTR by different mechanisms. Proceedings of the National Academy of Sciences of the United States of America. 2006;**103**(47):17891-17896

[9] Tavares B, Jacinto R, Sampaio P, Pestana S, Pinto A, Vaz A, et al. Notch/Her12 signalling modulates, motile/immotile cilia ratio downstream of Foxj1a in zebrafish left-right organizer. eLife. 2017;**6**:1-26

[10] Dasgupta A, Amack JD. Cilia in vertebrate left-right patterning. Philosophical Transactions of the Royal Society of London. Series B, Biological Sciences. 2016;**371**(1710):1-9

[11] Schottenfeld J, Sullivan-Brown J, Burdine RD. Zebrafish curly up encodes a Pkd2 ortholog that restricts left-side-specific expression of southpaw. Development. 2007;**134**(8):1605-1615

[12] Ferreira RR, Vilfan A, Jülicher F, Supatto W, Vermot J. Physical limits of flow sensing in the left-right organizer. eLife. 2017;**6**:1-27

[13] Wang G, Manning ML, Amack JD. Regional cell shape changes control form and function of Kupffer's vesicle in the zebrafish embryo. Developmental Biology. 2012;**370**(1):52-62

[14] Juan T, Géminard C, Coutelis JB, Cerezo D, Polès S, Noselli S, et al. Myosin1D is an evolutionarily conserved regulator of animal left-right asymmetry. Nature Communications. 2018;**9**(1):1942

[15] Compagnon J, Barone V, Rajshekar S, Kottmeier R, Pranjic-Ferscha K, Behrndt M, et al. The notochord breaks bilateral symmetry by controlling cell shapes in the zebrafish laterality organ. Developmental Cell. 2014;**31**(6):774-783

[16] Rubbo B, Lucas JS. Clinical care for primary ciliary dyskinesia: Current challenges and future directions. European Respiratory Review. 2017;**26**(145):1-11

[17] O'Callaghan C, Chetcuti P, Moya E. High prevalence of primary ciliary dyskinesia in a British Asian population. Archives of Disease in Childhood. 2010;**95**(1):51-52

[18] Loges NT, Antony D, Maver A, Deardorff MA, Güleç EY, Gezdirici A, et al. Recessive DNAH9 loss-of-function mutations cause laterality defects and subtle respiratory ciliary-beating defects. American Journal of Human Genetics. 2018;**103**(6):995-1008

[19] Ghandourah H, Dell SD. Severe disease due to CCDC40 gene variants and the perils of late diagnosis in primary ciliary dyskinesia. BML Case Reports. 2018;**2018**:bcr-2018-224964

[20] Rubbo B, Behan L, Dehlink E, Goutaki M, Hogg C, Kouis P, et al. Proceedings of the COST action BM1407 inaugural conference BEAT-PCD: Translational research in primary ciliary dyskinesia-bench, bedside, and population perspectives. BMC Proceedings. 2016;**10**(9):66

[21] Höben IM, Hjeij R, Olbrich H, Dougherty GW, Nöthe-Menchen T, Aprea I, et al. Mutations in C11orf70 cause primary ciliary dyskinesia with randomization of left/right body asymmetry due to defects of outer and inner dynein arms. American Journal of Human Genetics. 2018;**102**(5):973-984

[22] Olcese C, Patel MP, Shoemark A, Kiviluoto S, Legendre M, Williams HJ, et al. X-linked primary ciliary dyskinesia due to mutations in the cytoplasmic axonemal dynein assembly factor PIH1D3. Nature Communications. 2017;**8**:14279

[23] Cheong A, Degani R, Tremblay KD, Mager J. A null allele of Dnaaf2 displays embryonic lethality and mimics human ciliary dyskinesia. Human Molecular Genetics. 2019;**0**:1-10

[24] Afzelius BA. A human syndrome caused by immotile cilia. Science. 1976;**193**(4250):317-319

[25] Supp DM, Witte DP, Potter SS, Brueckner M. Mutation of an axonemal dynein affects left-right asymmetry in inversus viscerum mice. Nature. 1997;**389**(6654):963-966

[26] Nonaka S, Tanaka Y, Okada Y, Takeda S, Harada A, Kanai Y, et al. Randomization of left-right asymmetry due to loss of nodal cilia generating leftward flow of extraembryonic fluid in mice lacking KIF3B motor protein. Cell. 1998;**95**(6):829-837

[27] Nonaka S, Shiratori H, Saijoh Y, Hamada H. Determination of left-right patterning of the mouse embryo by artificial nodal flow. Nature. 2002;**418**(6893):96-99

[28] Norris DP, Grimes DT. Mouse models of ciliopathies: The state of the art. Disease Models & Mechanisms. 2012;**5**(3):299-312

[29] Grimes DT, Keynton JL, Buenavista MT, Jin X, Patel SH, Kyosuke S, et al. Genetic analysis reveals a hierarchy of interactions between polycystin-encoding genes and genes controlling cilia function during left-right determination. PLoS Genetics. 2016;**12**(6):e1006070

[30] Schweickert A, Weber T, Beyer T, Vick P, Bogusch S, Feistel K, et al. Cilia-driven leftward flow determines laterality in *Xenopus*. Current Biology. 2007;**17**(1):60-66

[31] Pintado P, Sampaio P, Tavares B, Montenegro-Johnson TD, Smith DJ, Lopes SS. Dynamics of cilia length in left-right development. Royal Society Open Science. 2017;**4**(3):161102

[32] Solowiej-Wedderburn J, Smith DJ, Lopes SS, Montenegro-Johnson TD. Wall stress enhanced exocytosis of extracellular vesicles as a possible mechanism of left-right symmetry-breaking in vertebrate development. Journal of Theoretical Biology. 2019;**460**:220-226

[33] Smith D, Montenegro-Johnson T, Lopes S. Organized chaos in Kupffer's vesicle: How a heterogeneous structure achieves consistent left-right patterning. BioArchitecture. 2014;**4**(3):119-125

[34] Okada Y, Nonaka S, Tanaka Y, Saijoh Y, Hamada H, Hirokawa N. Abnormal nodal flow precedes situs inversus in iv and inv mice. Molecular Cell. 1999;**4**(4):459-468

[35] McGrath J, Somlo S, Makova S, Tian X, Brueckner M. Two populations of node monocilia initiate left-right asymmetry in the mouse. Cell. 2003;**114**(1):61-73

[36] Tanaka Y, Okada Y, Hirokawa N. FGF-induced vesicular release of sonic hedgehog and retinoic acid in leftward nodal flow is critical for left-right determination. Nature. 2005;**435**(7039):172-177

[37] Neugebauer JM, Amack JD, Peterson AG, Bisgrove BW, Yost HJ. FGF signalling during embryo development regulates cilia length in diverse epithelia. Nature. 2009;**458**(7238):651-654

[38] Lopes SS, Lourenço R, Pacheco L, Moreno N, Kreiling J, Saúde L. Notch signalling regulates left-right asymmetry through ciliary length control. Development. 2010;**137**(21):3625-3632

[39] Kreiling JA, Prabhat, Williams G, Creton R. Analysis of Kupffer's vesicle in zebrafish embryos using a cave automated virtual environment. Developmental Dynamics 2007;236(7):1963-1969.

[40] Supatto W, Fraser SE, Vermot J. An all-optical approach for probing microscopic flows in living embryos. Biophysical Journal. 2008;**95**(4):L29-L31

[41] Yuan S, Zhao L, Brueckner M, Sun Z. Intraciliary calcium oscillations initiate vertebrate left-right asymmetry. Current Biology. 2015;**25**(5):556-567

[42] Willey CJ, Blais JD, Hall AK, Krasa HB, Makin AJ, Czerwiec FS. Prevalence of autosomal dominant polycystic kidney disease in the European Union. Nephrology, Dialysis, Transplantation. 2017;**32**(8):1356-1363

[43] Cornec-Le Gall E, Alam A, Perrone RD. Autosomal dominant polycystic kidney disease. Lancet. 2019;**393**(10174):919-935

[44] Porath B, Gainullin VG, Cornec-Le Gall E, Dillinger EK, Heyer CM, Hopp K, et al. Mutations in GANAB, encoding the glucosidase IIα subunit, cause autosomal-dominant polycystic kidney and liver disease. American Journal of Human Genetics. 2016;**98**(6):1193-1207

[45] Semmo M, Köttgen M, Hofherr A. The TRPP subfamily and polycystin-1 proteins. Handbook of Experimental Pharmacology. 2014;**222**:675-711

[46] Harris PC, Torres VE. Genetic mechanisms and signaling pathways in autosomal dominant polycystic kidney disease. The Journal of Clinical Investigation. 2014;**124**(6):2315-2324

[47] Torres VE, Harris PC. Strategies targeting cAMP signaling in the treatment of polycystic kidney disease. Journal of the American Society of Nephrology. 2014;**25**(1):18-32

[48] Horie S. Will introduction of tolvaptan change clinical practice in autosomal dominant polycystic kidney disease? Kidney International. 2015;**88**(1):14-16

[49] Reif GA, Yamaguchi T, Nivens E, Fujiki H, Pinto CS, Wallace DP. Tolvaptan inhibits ERK-dependent cell proliferation, Cl^- secretion, and in vitro cyst growth of human ADPKD cells stimulated by vasopressin. American Journal of Physiology. Renal Physiology. 2011;**301**(5):F1005-F1013

[50] Li H, Yang W, Mendes F, Amaral MD, Sheppard DN. Impact of the cystic fibrosis mutation F508del-CFTR on renal cyst formation and growth. American Journal of Physiology. Renal Physiology. 2012;**303**(8):F1176-F1186

[51] Yuajit C, Muanprasat C, Gallagher AR, Fedeles SV, Kittayaruksakul S, Homvisasevongsa S, et al. Steviol retards renal cyst growth through reduction of CFTR expression and inhibition of epithelial cell proliferation in a mouse model of polycystic kidney disease. Biochemical Pharmacology. 2014;**88**(3):412-421

[52] Yang B, Sonawane ND, Zhao D, Somlo S, Verkman AS. Small-molecule CFTR inhibitors slow cyst growth in polycystic kidney disease. Journal of the American Society of Nephrology. 2008;**19**(7):1300-1310

[53] Hanaoka K, Devuyst O, Schwiebert EM, Wilson PD, Guggino WB. A role for CFTR in human autosomal dominant polycystic kidney disease. The American Journal of Physiology. 1996;**270**(1):C389-C399

[54] Farinha CM, Matos P, Amaral MD. Control of cystic fibrosis transmembrane conductance regulator membrane trafficking: Not just from the endoplasmic reticulum to the Golgi. The FEBS Journal. 2013;**280**(18):4396-4406

[55] Lobo MJ, Amaral MD, Zaccolo M, Farinha CM. EPAC1 activation by cAMP stabilizes CFTR at the membrane by promoting its interaction with NHERF1. Journal of Cell Science. 2016;**129**(13):2599-2612

[56] Devuyst O, Chapman AB, Shoaf SE, Czerwiec FS, Blais JD. Tolerability of Aquaretic-related symptoms following Tolvaptan for autosomal dominant polycystic kidney disease: Results from TEMPO 3:4. Kidney International Reports. 2017;**2**(6):1132-1140

[57] De Rechter S, Breysem L, Mekahli D. Is autosomal dominant polycystic kidney disease becoming a pediatric disorder? Frontiers in Pediatrics. 2017;**5**:272

[58] Torres VE, Chapman AB, Devuyst O, Gansevoort RT, Grantham JJ, Higashihara E, et al. Tolvaptan in patients with autosomal dominant polycystic kidney disease. The New England Journal of Medicine. 2012;**367**(25):2407-2418

[59] England SJ, Campbell PC, Banerjee S, Swanson AJ, Lewis KE. Identification and expression analysis of the complete family of zebrafish pkd genes. Frontiers in Cell and Development Biology. 2017;**5**:5

[60] Mangos S, Lam PY, Zhao A, Liu Y, Mudumana S, Vasilyev A, et al. The ADPKD genes pkd1a/b and pkd2 regulate extracellular matrix formation. Disease Models & Mechanisms. 2010;**3**(5-6):354-365

[61] Obara T, Mangos S, Liu Y, Zhao J, Wiessner S, Kramer-Zucker AG, et al. Polycystin-2 immunolocalization and function in zebrafish. Journal of the American Society of Nephrology. 2006;**17**(10):2706-2718

[62] Sun Z, Amsterdam A, Pazour GJ, Cole DG, Miller MS, Hopkins N. A genetic screen in zebrafish identifies cilia genes as a principal cause of cystic kidney. Development. 2004;**131**(16):4085-4093

[63] Bisgrove BW, Snarr BS, Emrazian A, Yost HJ. Polaris and polycystin-2 in dorsal forerunner cells

and Kupffer's vesicle are required for specification of the zebrafish left-right axis. Developmental Biology. 2005;**287**(2):274-288

[64] Kamura K, Kobayashi D, Uehara Y, Koshida S, Iijima N, Kudo A, et al. Pkd1l1 complexes with Pkd2 on motile cilia and functions to establish the left-right axis. Development. 2011;**138**(6):1121-1129

[65] Thomson RB, Mentone S, Kim R, Earle K, Delpire E, Somlo S, et al. Histopathological analysis of renal cystic epithelia in the Pkd2WS25/− mouse model of ADPKD. American Journal of Physiology. Renal Physiology. 2003;**285**(5):F870-F880

[66] Cooper MS, Szeto DP, Sommers-Herivel G, Topczewski J, Solnica-Krezel L, Kang HC, et al. Visualizing morphogenesis in transgenic zebrafish embryos using BODIPY TR methyl ester dye as a vital counterstain for GFP. Developmental Dynamics. 2005;**232**(2):359-368

[67] Caron A, Xu X, Lin X. Wnt/β-catenin signaling directly regulates Foxj1 expression and ciliogenesis in zebrafish Kupffer's vesicle. Development. 2012;**139**(3):514-524

[68] Sakaguchi T, Kikuchi Y, Kuroiwa A, Takeda H, Stainier DY. The yolk syncytial layer regulates myocardial migration by influencing extracellular matrix assembly in zebrafish. Development. 2006;**133**(20):4063-4072

Chapter 4

Zebrafish as an Experimental Model for the Study of Obesity

Bárbara do Carmo Rodrigues Virote,
André Rodrigues da Cunha Barreto Vianna
and Luis David Solis Murgas

Abstract

Obesity is considered a silent global pandemic, with a steady increase in adults and children. It is a complex disease that involves the interaction of genetic and environmental factors and predisposes individuals to severe chronic complications such as various types of cancer, dyslipidemia, hyperglycemia, hypercholesterolemia, nonalcoholic fatty liver disease (NAFLD), and nonalcoholic steatohepatitis. To help elucidate the physiological mechanisms of this comorbidity in order to identify and develop effective treatments, the use of animal models is indispensable. Zebrafish is emerging as an important model for studying obesity and related metabolic diseases. In addition to being a small animal, with high genetic similarity when compared to humans and easy to handle, zebrafish also has the main well-conserved metabolism-related functions such as appetite regulation, insulin regulation, and lipid storage. Zebrafish is also suitable for the identification of new targets associated with the risk and treatment of obesity in humans. In this review, we highlight the studies that use zebrafish to study metabolic diseases demonstrating their important contribution in this area of research.

Keywords: metabolic syndrome, *Danio rerio*, transgenerationality, adiposity, inflammation

1. Introduction

The prevalence of obesity has increased significantly in the last three decades, being considered a pandemic that affects 1.9 billion people worldwide. In developed and developing countries, overweight and obesity are considered public health problems and have a high mortality rate due to associated risk factors [1].

Obesity is a risk factor for the development of type II diabetes mellitus (DM2), cardiovascular disease, hypertension, nonalcoholic liver disease, and cancer. Therefore, there is growing concern that it is estimated that the overall mortality rate from these non-transmissible diseases will increase in the coming decades [2].

Although it is a well-studied subject, many underlying biological mechanisms that mediate the effects of obesity are still unclear. Thus, animal models fill many of these gaps [3].

Zebrafish appears to be an excellent model for investigating the development of obesity, as it is a small fish, easy to maintain, and economical for breeding and has an easily observable and quantifiable behavior in a controlled environment [4]. In addition to these advantages of using zebrafish as a model, it still presents

IntechOpen

interesting features for studies of metabolic diseases such as organ conservation and physiology of energy metabolism [5].

Due to this ascendant use of zebrafish in this area of research, the objective of this work was to carry out a bibliographical review involving as a theme the use of zebrafish as an experimental model associated with obesity, demonstrating the advantages of using this model to study the mechanisms of metabolic diseases and characterization for new therapeutic targets in recent years.

2. The etiology of obesity

Obesity is defined as a heterogeneous biological disorder, having as one of the main contributors to the disease an unbalanced diet with the excessive intake of hypercaloric foods [6].

The extra calories ingested lead to the storage of excess nutrients in adipose cells, where they accumulate as triglycerides or neutral lipids [7]. This condition leads to an increase in adipose tissue, which can result in resistance to anorectic hormones such as insulin and leptin, and a change in the energy balance at the central level, characterized by decreased energy expenditure and increased food consumption [8].

One of the globally accepted indicators for diagnosing obesity is the body mass index (BMI) (weight/height^2). According to the most recent classification, an adult with a BMI value >25 kg/m^2 is considered overweight, and when this value is >30 kg/m^2, it is already treated as a degree of obesity [9].

With data reported in the last decades, many authors have already considered obesity as a global pandemic. This can be observed, for example, in a study conducted in 2015 showing that 107.7 million children and 603.7 million adults were obese worldwide. Among adults, the prevalence of obesity in 195 countries from 1980 to 2015 revealed a higher rate of obese women in all age groups, and for both sexes, the rate of increase in obesity was higher at the beginning of adulthood [10].

Obesity is not only a singular disorder but a multifactorial disease whose consequences are beyond the presentation of a characteristic phenotype [11]. The occurrence of obesity reflects the interaction of biological, behavioral, genetic, and environmental factors [12], which are associated with the development of severe chronic complications such as various types of cancer, dyslipidemia, hyperglycemia, hypercholesterolemia, nonalcoholic fatty liver disease, and nonalcoholic steatohepatitis [6].

Increased adiposity also causes a condition known as the metabolic syndrome, defined as a set of interrelated metabolic characteristics that are linked to the development of cardiovascular disease and diabetes [13]. To be considered as a syndrome, three of the following five factors are necessary for each individual: abdominal obesity (waist circumference ≥102 cm for men and ≥88 cm for women), high triglycerides, reduced high-density lipoprotein cholesterol, high arterial blood pressure, and altered fasting glycemia [14].

All these consequences of obesity occur, since the adipose tissue besides having the function of energy stock is also the largest endocrine organ of the human body [15]. Adipocytes are responsible for the production of substances that regulate various organic functions such as energy balance, secretion of peptides, bioactive proteins, and adipokines that are responsible for a series of metabolic alterations, such as in the control of food intake, in the control of insulin sensitivity, and in inflammatory processes [16].

In addition to being composed of adipocytes, adipose tissue is also composed of other types of cells, including lymphocytes, macrophages, fibroblasts, and vascular cells, which also play important roles in functional tissue control. Obesity generates large changes in the cellular composition of adipose tissue and also modulates the individual cell phenotype within this tissue [17]. Macrophages present two classes of known subpopulations: those with the capacity to produce pro-inflammatory cytokines, such as TNF-α, called M1, and those involved in anti-inflammatory reactions, expressing cytokines such as IL-10, called M2 [18]. In healthy individuals, macrophages are dispersed among adipocytes and, for the most part, constitute the M2 subtype. However, in obese individuals, monocytes tend to differentiate into M1 macrophages [19].

The exacerbated production of inflammatory signs by adipocytes that occurs in obese individuals stimulates the differentiation of M1 macrophages that in turn release nitric oxide, TNF-α, IL-6, and IL-1 [20]. These substances further stimulate the inflammatory activity of adipocytes. Thus, macrophages and adipocytes contribute, individually, to the inflammation state in adipose tissue, mutually stimulate each other's inflammatory activity, and contribute significantly to a chronic systemic inflammation of the obese individual [21].

In addition to metabolic disorders in the peripheral organs, inflammatory changes related to obesity also disrupt brain functions, especially affecting areas of the brain that regulate energy homeostasis and systemic metabolism [22].

The concern with obesity is increased by the fact that some data show that genes play an important role in predisposing individuals to obesity, showing that having one or both of the obese parents, especially the mother, increases the risk of obesity in the offspring [23]. Women who are overweight or obese when they enter pregnancy are more likely to have children more likely to develop obesity during childhood, adolescence, and adulthood [24]. This observed modulation not only happens with the maternal diet; researchers have identified epigenetic changes related to altered metabolism in the offspring resulting from variations in the father's diet, indicating that paternal behaviors may also put offspring at risk for obesity [25].

All these consequences show that nutritional status and diet are important factors related to the promotion and maintenance of good health. Obesity is one of the main causes of chronic non-transmissible diseases.

3. Zebrafish as a model for obesity

The regulation of energy expenditure and consumption involves many organs, including the brain, intestines, skeletal muscle, and adipose tissue. Therefore, the use of animal models is essential for a better understanding of the development and progression of metabolic dysfunction, such as obesity. Zebrafish is an excellent model for studying this type of disease because it has the major organs that are important for the regulation of energy homeostasis and metabolism in mammals including digestive organs, adipose tissue, and skeletal muscle. In addition, zebrafish has the main well-conserved functions, such as appetite regulation, insulin regulation, and lipid storage [5].

A primary characteristic of obesity is adipocyte hypertrophy and hyperplasia. Similar to mammalian white adipose tissue, adipocytes from the early-stage zebrafish contain several small lipid droplets, whereas mature adipocytes have a single large lipid droplet [26]. In zebrafish, lipids are also stored in visceral, intramuscular, and subcutaneous adipocytes [27], providing the opportunity to understand the regulation of body fat distribution in cases such as obesity.

The first diet-induced obese zebrafish model (DIO) was reported in 2010 through overfeeding with *Artemia* saline for 8 weeks. It has been shown through a comparative transcriptome analysis that the visceral adipose tissue between zebrafish, rat, mouse, and human has a similarity in lipid metabolism [28]. After the publication of Oka et al., several other methods of inducing obesity in zebrafish were applied as an induction by overfeeding with *Artemia* saline or commercial feed or through a hypercaloric diet with corn oil or commercial oil-enriched feed for different purposes of the study on obesity [7, 28–30].

Metabolic pathways that control body weight in mammals are conserved in the zebrafish. Therefore, zebrafish is often used as a transgenic model for obesity [5]. A note of caution is that not all genes of lipid metabolism are highly conserved in sequence and function in zebrafish. For example, zebrafish leptin protein is only 19% identical to human protein. In mice and humans, leptin is an adipostatic hormone that regulates adipose mass, and failure in leptin signaling results in hyperphagia and obesity [31]. Unlike mammals, leptin and leptin receptor are not expressed in adipose tissue in zebrafish. The zebrafish deficient in the leptin receptor has mainly interrupted glucose homeostasis [32], which is different from the phenotypes seen in mouse models such as severe hyperphagia, hyperlipidemia, and morbid obesity [33].

The zebrafish model presents important advantages over other models because it is a small fish, easy to maintain, and economical for breeding and has an easily observable and quantifiable behavior in a controlled environment [5]. The fact that it also has its sequenced genome and an extensive number of data in the literature facilitates the study of this model in the area on metabolic disorders such as obesity [34–36].

3.1 Modulating the processes of obesity

Obesity is dynamic; both its nature and its consequences are complex. This fact limits the decision-making process for the management of therapeutic options and prevention of the disease on a large scale, so the identification of the different pathways of induction to obesity is essential for subsequent studies.

As an example, there is a worrying fact that is gaining the attention of several researchers: the fact that obesity has a high prevalence in lower socioeconomic populations. Evidence shows that although genetic predisposition and a positive energy balance are implicated in obesity, environmental factors, including exposure to pesticides, heavy metals, and other contaminants, are widely suspected to have obesogenic activity, which are correlated with lower socioeconomic status [37, 38].

Zebrafish is also an excellent model for toxicological studies, and its use in this field of study has already demonstrated that the presence of cadmium in maternal blood during pregnancy is associated with an increased risk of juvenile obesity in offspring [37]. It has also been observed using zebrafish larvae that exposure to substances such as benzopyrene and ethanol may induce hepatotoxicity in vivo via membrane remodeling, leading to the condition of nonalcoholic fatty liver disease (NAFLD) that is closely linked to obesity [39].

In addition to uncovering this association between exposure to heavy metals and a higher incidence of obesity, zebrafish has been used to elucidate the modulation pathways of the influence of the microbiota on obesity. In recent decades it has been shown that intestinal microorganisms and diet represent attractive targets for controlling the absorption of dietary lipids and energy balance. Although the microbiota may influence nutrient uptake, diet may also affect the composition and function of the microbial community [40]. Recently, the profile of the intestinal microbiome in zebrafish with type 2 diabetes mellitus induced by obesity was performed. This work revealed functional similarities in intestinal bacterial environments between humans and zebrafish affected with DM2 [41].

Zebrafish is thus considered as an alternative model organism to study bacterial-host interactions in human obesity and related diseases. Thus, the zebrafish model becomes useful to uncover mechanisms that may respond, for example, to the efficiency of probiotics in modulating the microbiota, demonstrating whether they are capable of modifying host nutrient metabolism and energy homeostasis [42].

3.2 Drug screening and treatment

There is a recognized efficacy of the natural compounds combined with pharmacological treatment for the treatment of obesity, and thus there is a need to continually explore new anti-obesity compounds [43].

Within this scope, the zebrafish is a model with upward relevance for the discovery of new drugs for metabolic disturbances. The advantage of the use of this model for the screening of new drugs is due to the fact that zebrafish is already consecrated for preclinical tests.

In the larval stage, zebrafish is used to identify nontoxic molecules to treat obesity, since at that stage they already have those of signal transduction pathways that regulate lipid metabolism [44]. Another example is the use of zebrafish transgenic larvae expressing GFP on neutrophils, which allows visualization of recruitment of neutrophils to a specific site injured, in vivo and in real time. This model has been widely characterized in the last 10 years, demonstrating the conservation of cellular and molecular mechanisms with inflammatory processes in mammals and allowing the discovery and testing of anti-inflammatory compounds that have mechanisms closely related to obesity [45].

About work performed in adulthood, when used to study the development of type 2 diabetes mellitus through overfeeding, zebrafish has been shown to have human-like responses to antidiabetic drugs such as metformin and glibenclamide. In this way, the zebrafish was shown to be a suitable model also for identifying therapeutic targets and chemical screening in that area [29].

Research has also been conducted using the zebrafish model to evidence the effect of green tea extract, *Camellia sinensis*, in inhibiting lipid accumulation, decreasing the volume of visceral adipose tissue, and altering the expression of catabolic lipid genes [30]. On the other hand, other studies have demonstrated the effect and mechanisms of β-glucan derived from the edible fungus, *Agaricus bisporus*, regulating lipid metabolism and preventing lipid deposition and providing experimental data for its use in diet and food dependence [46]. It is also observed that the use of a natural polyphenol, resveratrol, has anti-obesity effects via regulation of lipid metabolism [47].

In recent studies the use of zebrafish for the study of secondary metabolites with bioactivities relevant to various metabolic functions produced by marine cyanobacteria was observed and some substances with activities of significant reduction of lipids [48, 49].

In addition to studies for the identification of new drugs, zebrafish is also used to elucidate the mechanisms underlying the effect of certain known substances. As an example, it has been reported that the substance tanshinone IIA has anti-adipogenic and anti-obesity effects on 3T3-L1 cells in obese mice induced by hypercaloric diet; however the mechanisms for this condition were little known. With the use of zebrafish that demonstrated the same response to the substance tanshinone IIA, it was observed that the anti-adipogenic effect of tanshinone IIA in 3T3-L1 cells is mediated by the control of the expression and/or phosphorylation levels of C/EBP-α, PPAR-γ, FAS, perilipin A, and STAT-3/5 [50].

As the consolidation of zebrafish for the study of obesity was recently performed, it is still a poorly studied model and has great potential to be explored in several areas of study on the metabolic syndrome and discovery of new therapeutic targets.

4. Conclusions

Knowing the problems caused by obesity and its alarming increase, it was observed in this review that many mechanisms underlying this condition have not yet been elucidated. It has also been shown that zebrafish is emerging as a relevant model in the study of obesity and related metabolic disorders. The advantages that make zebrafish a more adequate model when compared to other animals, such as rodents, are associated with its good efficacy to characterize the mechanisms and pathways involved in diseases, its ability to test new pharmacological and therapeutic approaches, the need for small amounts of compost for drug testing, low cost of maintenance, and conservation of the main metabolic pathways related to energy status. In this sense, zebrafish appears as a relevant model for preclinical trials and shows to be a model with great potential to help solve problems related to obesity.

Acknowledgements

The authors gratefully acknowledge the financial support of the Conselho Nacional de Desenvolvimento Científico e Tecnológico (CNPq), the Coordenação de Aperfeiçoamento de Nível Superior (CAPES), and the Fundação de Amparo à Pesquisa do Estado de Minas Gerais (FAPEMIG).

Conflict of interest

None of the authors have any conflicts of interest.

Author details

Bárbara do Carmo Rodrigues Virote[1], André Rodrigues da Cunha Barreto Vianna[2] and Luis David Solis Murgas[1*]

1 Federal University of Lavras, Lavras, Brazil

2 Federal University of Paraná, Palotina, Brazil

*Address all correspondence to: lsmurgas@ufla.br

References

[1] Freitas W, Oliveira L, Perez E, Ilias E, Lottenberg B, Silva A, et al. Systemic inflammation in severe obese patients undergoing surgery for obesity and weight-related diseases. Obesity Surgery. 2018;**28**:1931-1942. DOI: 10.1007/s11695-017-3104-9

[2] Schlegel A, Gut P. Metabolic insights from zebrafish genetics, physiology, and chemical biology. Cellular and Molecular Life Sciences. 2015;**72**:2249-2260. DOI: 10.1007/s00018-014-1816-8

[3] Baker T, Peterson R, Heideman W. Using zebrafish as a model system for studying the transgenerational effects of dioxin. Toxicological Sciences. 2014;**138**:403-411. DOI: 10.1093/toxsci/kfu006

[4] Spence R, Gerlach G, Lawrence C, Smith C. The behaviour and ecology of the zebrafish, *Danio rerio*. Biological Reviews of the Cambridge Philosophical Society. 2008;**83**:13-34. DOI: 10.1111/j.1469-185X.2007.00030.x

[5] Zang L, Maddison A, Chen W. Zebrafish as a model for obesity and diabetes. Frontiers in Cell and Development Biology. 2018;**6**:91. DOI: 10.3389/fcell.2018.00091

[6] World Health Organization (WHO). Diet, nutrition and the prevention of chronic diseases. Report of a joint WHO/FAO expert consultation. Available from: http://apps.who.int/iris/bitstream/10665/42665/1/WHO_TRS_916.pdf [Accessed: 20 June 2019]

[7] Vargas R, Vásquez I. Mint: Effects of overfeeding and high-fat diet on cardiosomatic parameters and cardiac structures in young and adult zebrafish. Fish Physiology and Biochemistry. 2017;**43**:1761-1773. DOI: 10.1007/s10695-017-0407-7

[8] Barreto-Vianna A, Aguila B, Mandarim-De-Lacerda A. Effects of liraglutide in hypothalamic arcuate nucleus of obese mice. Obesity. 2016;**24**:626-633. DOI: 10.1002/oby.21387

[9] Seidell C, Halberstadt J. The global burden of obesity and the challenges of prevention. Annals of Nutrition and Metabolism. 2015;**66**:7-12. DOI: 10.1159/000375143

[10] GBD 2015 Obesity Collaborators. Health effects of overweight and obesity in 195 countries over 25 years. The New England Journal of Medicine. 2017;**377**:13-27. DOI: 10.1056/NEJMoa1614362

[11] Brito AKP. Relação entre a microbiota intestinal, níveis de grelina e leptina e perfil inflamatório de mulheres eutróficas e obesas [thesis]. Bahia: Federal University of Bahia; 2018

[12] Lee B, Bartsch S, Mui Y, Haidari L, Spiker M, Gittelsohn J. A systems approach to obesity. Nutrition Reviews. 2017;**75**:94-106. DOI: 10.1093/nutrit/nuw049

[13] Grundy S, Brewer H Jr, Cleeman J, SmithJr S, Lenfante C. Definition of metabolic syndrome: Report of the National Heart, Lung, and Blood Institute/American Heart Association conference on scientific issues related to definition. Circulation. 2004;**109**:433-438. DOI: 10.1161/01

[14] Expert Panel On Detection, Evaluation et al. Executive summary of the third report of the National Cholesterol Education Program (NCEP) expert panel on detection, evaluation, and treatment of high blood cholesterol in adults (adult treatment panel III). JAMA. 2001;**285**:2486. DOI: 10.1001/jama.285.19.2486

[15] Orio F, Muscogiuri G, Nesse C, Palomba Savastano S, Tafuri D, Colariete G, et al. Obesity, type 2 diabetes mellitus and cardiovascular disease risk: An uptodate in the management of polycystic ovary syndrome. European Journal of Obstetrics, Gynecology, and Reproductive Biology. 2016;**207**:214-219. DOI: 10.1016/j.ejogrb.2016.08.026

[16] Fichman V. Investigando a associação da obesidade com a infertilidade [thesis]. Rio de Janeiro: Foundation Oswaldo Cruz; 2018

[17] Nakamura K, Fuster J, Walsh K. Adipokines: A link between obesity and cardiovascular disease. Journal of Cardiology. 2014;**63**:250-259. DOI: 10.1016/j.jjcc.2013.11.006

[18] Lumeng C, Bodzin JL, Saltiel AR. O besity induces a phenotypic switch in adipose tissue macrophage polarization. The Journal of Clinical Investigation. 2007;**117**:175-184. DOI: 10.1172/JCI29881

[19] de Almeida LB. Efeito da obesidade pré-gestacional no teor de citocinas de compartimentos maternos e fetais e na expressão de transportadores de ácidos graxos da placenta [thesis]. Rio de Janeiro: Federal University of Rio de Janeiro; 2017

[20] Weisberg S, McCann D, Desai M, Rosenbaum M, Leibel R, Ferrante A Jr. Obesity is associated with macrophage accumulation in adipose tissue. Journal of Clinical Investigation. 2003;**112**: 1796-1808. DOI: 10.1172/JCI19246

[21] Berg H, Scherer E. Adipose tissue, inflammation, and cardiovascular disease. Circulation Research. 2005;**96**:939-949. DOI: 10.1161/01

[22] Jais A, Brüning J. Hypothalamic inflammation in obesity and metabolic disease. Journal of Clinical Investigation. 2017;**127**:24-32. DOI: 10.1172/JCI88878

[23] Maffeis C, Morandi A. Effect of maternal obesity on foetal growth and metabolic health of the offspring. Obesity Facts. 2017;**10**:112-117. DOI: 10.1159/000456668

[24] Haire-Joshu D, Tabak R. Preventing obesity across generations: Evidence for early life intervention. Annual Review of Public Health. 2016;**37**:253-271. DOI: 10.1146/annurev-publhealth-032315-021859

[25] Ozanne S. Epigenetic signatures of obesity. The New England Journal of Medicine. 2015;**372**:973-974. DOI: 10.1056/NEJMcibr1414707

[26] Flynn E, Trent C, Rawls J. Ontogeny and nutritional control of adipogenesis in zebrafish (*Danio rerio*). Journal of Lipid Research. 2009;**50**:1641-1652. DOI: 10.1194/jlr.M800590-JLR200

[27] Song Y, Cone D. Creation of a genetic model of obesity in a teleost. The FASEB Journal. 2007;**21**:2042-2049. DOI: 10.1096/fj.06-7503com

[28] Oka T, Nishimura Y, Zang L, Hirano M, Shimada Y, Wang Z, et al. Diet-induced obesity in zebrafish shares common pathophysiological pathways with mammalian obesity. BMC Physiology. 2010;**10**:21. DOI: 10.1186/1472-6793-10-21

[29] Zang L, Shimada Y, Nishimura N. Development of a novel zebrafish model for type 2 diabetes mellitus. Scientific Reports. 2017;**1**:1461. DOI: 10.1038/s41598-017-01432-w

[30] Meguro S, Hasumura T, Hase T. Body fat accumulation in zebrafish is induced by a diet rich in fat and reduced by supplementation with green tea extract. PLoS ONE. 2015;**10**:0120142. DOI: 10.1371/journal.pone.0120142

[31] Myers M Jr, Leibel R, Seeley R, Schwartz M. Obesity and leptin resistance: Distinguishing cause

from effect. Trends in Endocrinology and Metabolism. 2010;**21**:643-651. DOI: 10.1016/j.tem.2010.08.002

[32] Michel M, Page-McCaw P, Chen W, Cone R. Leptin signaling regulates glucose homeostasis, but not adipostasis, in the zebrafish. Proceedings of the National Academy of Sciences. 2016;**113**:3084-3089. DOI: 10.1073/pnas.1513212113

[33] Inagaki-Ohara K. Gastric leptin and tumorigenesis: Beyond obesity. International Journal of Molecular Sciences. 2622;**2019**:20. DOI: 10.3390/ijms20112622

[34] Garcia G, Noyes P, Tanguay R. Advancements in zebrafish applications for 21st century toxicology. Pharmacology and Therapeutics. 2016;**161**:11-21. DOI: 10.1016/j.pharmthera.2016.03.009

[35] Hoo J, Kumari Y, Shaikh M, Hue S, Goh B. Zebrafish: A versatile animal model for fertility research. BioMed Research International. 2016;**2016**:20. DOI: 10.1155/2016/9732780

[36] Chakraborty C, Sharma A, Sharma G, Lee S. Zebrafish: A complete animal model to enumerate the nanoparticle toxicity. Journal of Nanobiotechnology. 2016;**14**:65. DOI: 10.1186/s12951-016-0217-6

[37] Green A, Hoyo C, Mattlingy C, Luo Y, Tzeng J, Murphy S, et al. Cadmium exposure increases the risk of juvenile obesity: A human and zebrafish comparative study. International Journal of Obesity. 2018;**42**:1285-1295. DOI: 10.1038/s41366-018-0036-y

[38] Planchart A, Green A, Hoyo C, Mattlingy C. Heavy metal exposure and metabolic syndrome: Evidence from human and model system studies. Current Environmental Health Reports. 2018;**5**:110-124. DOI: 10.1007/s40572-018-0182-3

[39] Imran M, Sergent O, Tête A, Gallais I, Chevanne M, Lagadic-Gossmann D, et al. Membrane remodeling as a key player of the hepatotoxicity induced by co-exposure to benzo[a]pyrene and ethanol of obese zebrafish larvae. Biomolecules. 2018;**8**:26. DOI: 10.3390/biom8020026

[40] Semova I, Carten J, Stombaugh J, Mackey L, Knight R, Farber S, et al. Microbiota regulate intestinal absorption and metabolism of fatty acids in the zebrafish. Cell Host & Microbe. 2012;**12**:277-288. DOI: 10.1016/j.chom.2012.08.003

[41] Okazaki F, Zang L, Nakayama H, Chen Z, Gao Z, Chiba H, et al. Microbiome alteration in type 2 diabetes mellitus model of zebrafish. Scientific Reports. 2019;**9**:867. DOI: 10.1038/s41598-018-37242-x

[42] Falcinelli S, Rodiles A, Hatef A, Picchietti S, Cossignani L, Merrifield D, et al. Dietary lipid content reorganizes gut microbiota and probiotic *L. rhamnosus* attenuates obesity and enhances catabolic hormonal milieu in zebrafish. Scientific Reports. 2017;7:5512. DOI: 10.1038/s41598-017-05147-w

[43] Lee H, Li H, Kweon M, Choi Y, Kim M, Ryu J. Isobavachalcone from Angelica keiskei inhibits adipogenesis and prevents lipid accumulation. International Journal of Molecular Sciences. 2018;**19**:1693. DOI: 10.3390/ijms19061693

[44] Jones K, Alimov A, Rilo H, Jandacek R, Woollet L, Penberthy W. A high throughput live transparent animal bioassay to identify non-toxic small molecules or genes that regulate vertebrate fat metabolism for obesity drug development. Nutrition and Metabolism. 2008;**5**:23. DOI: 10.1186/1743-7075-5-23

[45] Rodriguez-Duarte J, Dapueto R, Galliussi G, Turell L, Kamaid A. Electrophilic

nitroalkene-tocopherol derivatives: Synthesis, physicochemical characterization and evaluation of anti-inflammatory signaling responses. Scientific Reports. 2018;**8**:12784. DOI: 10.1038/s41598-018-31218-7

[46] Li X, Xue Y, Pang L, Len B, Lin Z, Huang J, et al. Agaricus bisporus-derived β-glucan prevents obesity through PPAR γ downregulation and autophagy induction in zebrafish fed by chicken egg yolk. International Journal of Biological Macromolecules. 2019;**125**:820-828. DOI: 10.1016/j.ijbiomac.2018.12.122

[47] Ran G, Ying L, Li L, Yan Q, Yi W, Ying C, et al. Resveratrol ameliorates diet-induced dysregulation of lipid metabolism in zebrafish (*Danio rerio*). PLoS ONE. 2017;**12**:0180865. DOI: 10.1371/journal.pone.0180865

[48] Costa M, Rosa F, Ribeiro T, Hernandez-Bautista R, Bonaldo M, Silva N, et al. Identification of cyanobacterial strains with potential for the treatment of obesity-related co-morbidities by bioactivity toxicity evaluation and metabolite profiling. Marine Drugs. 2019;**17**:280. DOI: 10.3390/md17050280

[49] Freitas S, Silva N, Souza M, Ribeiro T, Rosa F, Leão P, et al. Chlorophyll derivatives from marine cyanobacteria with lipid-reducing activities. Marine Drugs. 2019;**17**:229. DOI: 10.3390/md17040229

[50] Park Y, Obiang-Obounou B, Lee J, Lee T, Bae M, Hwang K, et al. Anti-adipogenic effects on 3t3-l1 cells and zebrafish by tanshinone IIA. International Journal of Molecular Sciences. 2017;**18**:2065. DOI: 10.3390/ijms18102065

Section 4

Using of Zebrafish in Toxicology and Drug Development

Chapter 5

Histopathology of Zebrafish (*Danio rerio*) in Nonclinical Toxicological Studies of New Drugs

Raphaelle Sousa Borges, Arlindo César Matias Pereira, Gisele Custodio de Souza and José Carlos Tavares Carvalho

Abstract

Zebrafish (*Danio rerio*) is a small-sized teleost fish natural of tropical regions, with a short life cycle and high homology toward humans. These features make zebrafish an attractive and promising model organism for nonclinical tests due to the ease of handling and cost–benefit compared to other models. The digestive, cardiovascular, urinary, nervous, and reproductive systems of zebrafish display feature similar to those of superior mammals, and due to its susceptible organs, the adult zebrafish has been used to test the toxicity of environmental compounds and potential drug candidates through histopathology analysis complementarily with other parameters. In such cases, the choice of the organ assessed relies on the type of compound tested, administration route, and biological activity. This chapter brings together histopathological nonclinical toxicity studies performed exclusively with zebrafish, highlighting significant histological changes found in its gills, liver, kidneys, and intestine. Based on the information presented here, it is expected that the researcher recognizes differences between healthy and changed tissue, without having to compare its result with other species.

Keywords: preclinical, histopathology, drug development, histology, zebrafish

1. Introduction

Zebrafish (*Danio rerio*) is a teleost fish from the family Cyprinidae, inhabiting fresh water of tropical regions. It is natural of Bangladesh, Nepal, and India and is popularly sold as an ornamental fish [1]. It has a small size and reaches up to 5 centimeters of length. The species often adapts to environmental changes of temperature and pH.

Since the first use of zebrafish as an experimental model in 1955, it has been consolidated as a model organism for biology, genetics, pharmacology, and general biomedical research. The exponential growth of zebrafish use in laboratories is due to several favorable features such as its fast life cycle (the adult stage reached about 6 months), high fecundity (hundreds of eggs are laid in each mating), transparency of the embryonic/larval stages which facilitates the observation of the development, low maintenance cost, and easy handling [2]. Due to its small size and low body weight, it requires a relatively low quantity of the compound tested, which is an excellent advantage in the research [3]. Despite the phylogenetic distance, zebrafish has about 70% of genetic homology toward humans [4]; hence, it is considered a reliable tool for preclinical studies.

In pharmacology, determining the toxicity of the tested compound is a crucial step in preclinical studies since it will be the base for clinical trials when it is tested in humans. Zebrafish has been gaining attention for toxicological assays, either of administered compounds or those present in the environment due to its physiological response and histological features similar of those of mammals, potentially reducing the number of rodents used in the laboratory routine [2]. The sensibility of zebrafish organs to harmful compounds makes it possible to appraise through histopathology the safety of potentially bioactive substances [5]. Therefore, tissue changes are a useful tool to assess how a tested compound can exert a toxic in the animal; for this, it is essential to choose the most appropriate organs to be assessed [6].

The major organs accountable to metabolize and excrete xenobiotics are the liver and the kidney. The liver of zebrafish has disorganized hepatocytes and lacks Kupffer cells accountable to phagocyte foreign bodies [7]. However, despite these structural divergences, there are conserved aspects compared to the liver of mammals, for instance, the presence of hepatocytes and their main physiological processes performed through the action of the cytochrome P450, which makes it possible to compare hepatic lesions caused by nocive compounds in humans [8].

The kidneys have lymphoid, endocrine, and hematopoietic tissues. The latter is accountable to perform the functions of the bone marrow, absent in zebrafish. The renal filtration process contributes to the excretion of compounds previously metabolized in the liver. In zebrafish, both renal function and the glomeruli structure are similar to mammals, enabling the comparison of histopathology [9].

Zebrafish is an ideal model to assess environmental toxicity [10]. In these studies, the potentially toxic compounds present in the water are rapidly absorbed through the gills. Hence, the gills are an essential organ to perform histopathology when the fish absorb the compounds through immersion. Besides performing gas exchanges, the gills have a crucial role in the maintenance of osmotic balance, excretion of nitrogenated compounds, and acid–base balance of the adult fish.

The gastrointestinal tract of zebrafish, like those of mammals, has a mucous layer of simple columnar epithelial tissue formed by enterocytes arranged around the villi. Despite not having a stomach, the intestinal bulb—anterior portion of the intestine—substitutes this organ in its functions such as nutrient digestion and absorption. Therefore, histopathology of the intestine can be a useful tool to assess the safety of orally administered compounds [5]. Another difference compared to the gastrointestinal tract of mammals is the lack of Paneth cells and crypts of Lieberkuhn.

In the literature, the morphology of healthy zebrafish tissues is well known. However, to date, there are few studies dedicated exclusively to the comparison between healthy zebrafish and changed histopathology of the major organs of excretion and metabolization. Hence, this chapter aims to fill this gap in the literature, providing material for the researcher to better understand the histopathology of these organs in zebrafish, without needing to compare its results with other species. Also, the reader will learn the significant similarities and differences of zebrafish tissues compared to mammals, which is essential to interpret its results adequately.

2. Histopathology as a tool to assess toxicity in adult zebrafish

The potential of a chemical compound to induce injury to an organism is called toxicity. The toxic action depends on several factors such as the period of exposure, mechanisms of transport, and target site interaction. One way to understand the effect of chemical agents in a living organism is the toxicity assays [11]. Toxicity assays are a critical step in the preclinical evaluation of new drugs; also, they are performed in environmental toxicity assessment of pollutants. For this, it is necessary to employ animal models able to extrapolate the results to humans posteriorly; hence, the animal chosen must have defined similarities with them, such as in the tissues and physiological response.

The study of tissue alterations is defined as histopathology. This method is useful to detect potentially deleterious effects of compounds to a particular organ or tissue [6]. The choice of the organ depends on the type of compound tested and the metabolism of the animal used. Zebrafish is an excellent model to perform histopathology assessment [12]. The genetic homology and conserved aspects compared to humans can be extended to disease phenotypes to perform comparisons [2]. Several organs of zebrafish have been used in toxicological studies, such as the gonads, pharynx, thyroid, intestine, liver, kidney, gills, and muscles. A considerable advantage of zebrafish in histopathology is the possibility to observe several organs in only one slide due to its small size.

Histopathology of zebrafish gonads was capable of showing the detrimental effects of chronic treatment of bezafibrate in gonad steroidogenesis and spermatogenesis. The bezafibrate—drug used in the control of cholesterol levels in humans—was administered orally in male zebrafish. The histological analysis showed testicular degeneration, and this could improve our understanding of the possible risks of prolonged bezafibrate use in the reduction of fertility in humans [13].

The gonads were also used to evaluate the long period of treatment with the hydroethanolic extract from *Acmella oleracea*, the "jambú," in adult zebrafish. This plant is popular in cooking from the north of Brazil and is used as an aphrodisiac agent. The results showed low toxicity, evidenced by few tissue changes in the ovaries and testes [14].

The muscle of zebrafish was used to perform histopathological analysis on the toxicity of *Streptomyces* sp. AKS2, a potential antibacterial against *Klebsiella* sp., injected intramuscularly. The tissue did not have changes, suggesting low toxicity. This study could point further uses of the muscle histopathology in future toxicity assays [15].

Despite often used to assess the effect of chemical compounds in the endocrine system, the histopathology of the thyroid has been reported less in fish models. Schmidt et al. [15] reported that sublethal concentrations of propylthiouracil and perchlorate induced cell changes in the thyrocytes, evidencing the efficacy of zebrafish thyroid tissue histopathology in toxicity assays. Moreover, histopathology analysis of thyroid tissue in male zebrafish was essential to assess the toxic effect of prolonged exposure to fluoride in this organ [16].

The gills are crucial to assess the toxicity of chemical compounds suspended in the water in environmental toxicity studies. Female zebrafish had few tissue alterations in the gills when exposed to silver nanoparticles [16]. However, in the presence of uranium, the gills, gonads, and muscles were affected, demonstrating the dangers of the contamination with this element [17].

In a study assessing the toxic effects of thallium—chemical element emitted mainly after combustion of mineral coal, easily incorporated to the soil and water—the gills were injured even at the lowest concentrations [18]. In another study, zebrafish exposed to cobalt chloride showed relevant tissue alterations in the gills, pharynx, and intestinal mucosa. The authors stated that adult zebrafish could provide a robust model to assess indicators of toxicity from chemical products [19]. Overall, these studies indicate that the histopathology of zebrafish gills can be a reliable model to assess whether a chemical compound is toxic.

As for the liver, there are relevant similarities between the liver of zebrafish and those of superior mammals in the most basal aspects and regulatory mechanisms related to hepatoxicity [19]. Due to its role in animals, the liver is essential to assess the metabolism of xenobiotic compounds.

Chronic administration of the fungicide boscalid induced histological injury in liver and kidney of zebrafish, hampering the metabolism of carbohydrates and lipids and the healthy development of the animals [20]. Moreover, in a study in which the fishes were exposed to tris(1,3-dichloro-2-propyl)phosphate (TDCPP), the liver of the animals had increased size and tissue alterations, showing the sensibility of this organ and its role in detoxification [21].

After subacute exposure to pharmaceutical products—such as carbamazepine, fenofibric acid, propranolol, sulfamethoxazole, and trimethoprim—the tissue changes in the liver varied according to the sex, being more prevalent in male fishes, whose the liver tended to increase and have more tissue alteration, reinforcing the importance of controlling the sexes in toxicological studies [22].

The females also can be used; in a study using female zebrafish exposed to sodium fluoride (NaF), the fishes had tissue degeneration [22]. In another study, long-term exposure to perfluorooctane sulfonate (PFOS) induced accumulation of lipid droplets in the liver of males and inhibited the growth of the gonads of female zebrafishes, suggesting a potential to induce malformation in embryos from exposed fishes [23].

The kidney and intestine have a role in the excretion of substances and are valuable to assess the toxicity of them. For instance, the intestine of adult zebrafish was used to assess the impact of silver nanoparticles coated with citrate [24] and cadmium present in the environment [25]. In the latter, the results showed a nonlinear response to the toxic effects, suggesting that the animals used may have developed a defense mechanism against the toxicity related to hormesis.

A method to quantify the tissue changes in zebrafish organs is through the histological alteration index (HAI). This method takes into consideration the average tissue changes based on a list of possible changes classified into three levels of severity. The method was first conceived for gills and, posteriorly, was adapted to the liver, kidney, and intestine, due to their sensibility to injuries caused by toxic agents [5, 9, 16, 26].

3. Main histological changes found in zebrafish organs after exposure to toxic compounds

In this section the major tissue changes caused by potentially toxic compounds observed in the gills, liver, kidney, and intestine and the possible physiological response that cause them will be presented. Pictures will be shown to compare healthy and changed tissues.

3.1 Gills

Zebrafish has four gill arches in each side of the pharynx; each of them has two rows of filaments, which in turn has secondary lamellae in both sides [11]. Firstly, the water enters through the oral cavity; then, it passes through the pharynx and gills, where the gas exchange occurs. The water is pushed through contraction and relaxation of the vestibular muscle and the operculum movements. The primary lamellae (gill filaments) are in the central portion of the gills formed by cartilaginous tissue supporting the venous sinusoids [7, 27].

Besides being accountable to perform the gas exchange in the water, the gills also have a role in the excretion of residues [27]. This organ is highly sensitive to toxic compounds, and when exposed to them, it has typical tissue changes. One of the first alterations observed is the displacement of the lamella epithelial cells, which, according to Carvalho et al. [5], can indicate an adaptation attempt in the aquatic animal to the ongoing new environmental conditions. The space between the lamellae and the displaced epithelial tissue is filled with water, forming edema, which can hamper the function of this organ, suffocating the animal [28].

The change in the function of the gills can lead to an increase in size in the epithelial cells (hyperplasia). As a consequence of hyperplasia, the fusion of secondary lamellae can occur [29]. This feature blocks the passage of water and blood to decrease the work overload of lamellae cells. However, it causes a deficit of oxygenation and can induce the death of the animal [30].

Chloride cells are located on the basis of secondary lamellae and are accountable to pump sodium and chloride ions into the fish to maintain its osmotic balance [27].

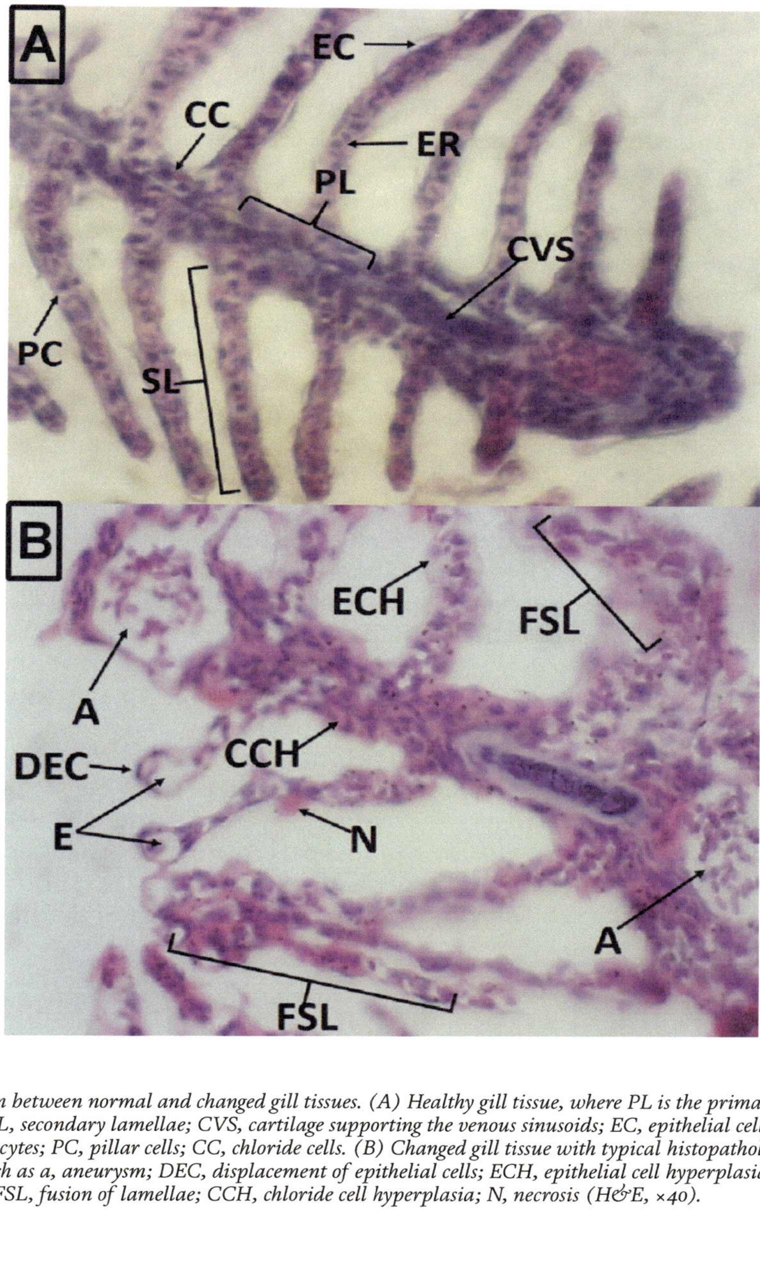

Figure 1.
Comparison between normal and changed gill tissues. (A) Healthy gill tissue, where PL is the primary lamellae; SL, secondary lamellae; CVS, cartilage supporting the venous sinusoids; EC, epithelial cells; ER, erythrocytes; PC, pillar cells; CC, chloride cells. (B) Changed gill tissue with typical histopathological changes, such as a, aneurysm; DEC, displacement of epithelial cells; ECH, epithelial cell hyperplasia; E, edema; FSL, fusion of lamellae; CCH, chloride cell hyperplasia; N, necrosis (H&E, ×40).

Hence, hyperplasia in these cells may indicate an osmotic imbalance in the fish, as the organism tries to adapt through the increase of sodium and chloride transport into the blood to reestablish the homeostasis [31].

Another essential cell in the maintenance of blood circulation is the pillar cell. Changes in its regular function can induce lamellae degeneration and blood flow dysregulation [32]. Progressive distension of the pillar cells can cause aneurysms, hemorrhages, and gill tissue collapse through all lamellae [5]. High toxicity-induced cell degeneration in the lamellae causes loss of tissue function, and hence, if necrosis is observed, the dose of the compound tested is highly toxic. Healthy gill tissue and significant tissue changes caused by toxic compounds cited in this section are shown in **Figure 1**.

3.2 Liver

The hepatocytes are the primary cells of the zebrafish liver and form the hepatic cords. In zebrafish—like in superior mammals—these cells act in the processing of proteins, carbohydrates, lipids, and vitamins and detoxification of xenobiotic compounds. The hepatocytes are accountable to synthesize the bile, which is transported through the bile ducts. Blood vessels are frequent and abundant in the liver [7, 27].

A common tissue alteration found in the hepatocytes is cytoplasm vacuolization due to a decrease of glycogen stores and lipid accumulation, which could be due to the action of toxic agents. This process is believed to hamper the normal function of the liver [9]. However, the decrease of glycogen stores should not be considered alone since due to the small size and high agility of zebrafish, zebrafish has an accelerated metabolism which can consume the glycogen if the animal is active enough [5, 29].

Changes in the nuclei morphology, such as vacuolization and atrophy, are often observed when functional alterations occur in the hepatocytes and can precede pyknosis (reduction and rounding of the nuclei that precedes apoptosis) and cellular degeneration. On the other hand, hypertrophy of the nuclei indicates intense metabolic activity in the hepatocytes, which can be caused by exposure to toxic agents [33]. When the hepatocytes degenerate, a relative reduction in the frequency of nuclei is observed, which is believed to be a defense mechanism.

The bile excretion also can be affected by toxic agents, causing cholestasis, which is an indication of liver dysfunction. Histopathologically, this is detected through the presence of brownish pigment inside the cells and is attributed to the failure in the excretion of bile pigments due to decreased capacity of bonding between bilirubin and glucuronic acid [29].

Other frequent changes observed are the increased frequency of blood vessels and hyperemia, mechanisms triggered to increase the blood flow to the liver, consequently increasing the supply of oxygen and nutrients in the affected area, preventing hypoxia [5, 9, 33]. Finally, if the animals are exposed to high levels of a toxic agent, rupture of blood vessels and tissue necrosis can occur. The tissue changes of the liver cited in the section and the normal histology of the organ are shown in **Figure 2**.

3.3 Kidneys

The kidney of zebrafish is accountable to excrete the excess of water that enters through the mouth; it also has a role in the filtration of residues and osmotic balance [9, 27]. This organ is one of the most affected by toxic compounds and has conserved similarities compared to those of mammals [5]. The nephrons are formed by glomeruli and distal and proximal tubules; the glomeruli are surrounded

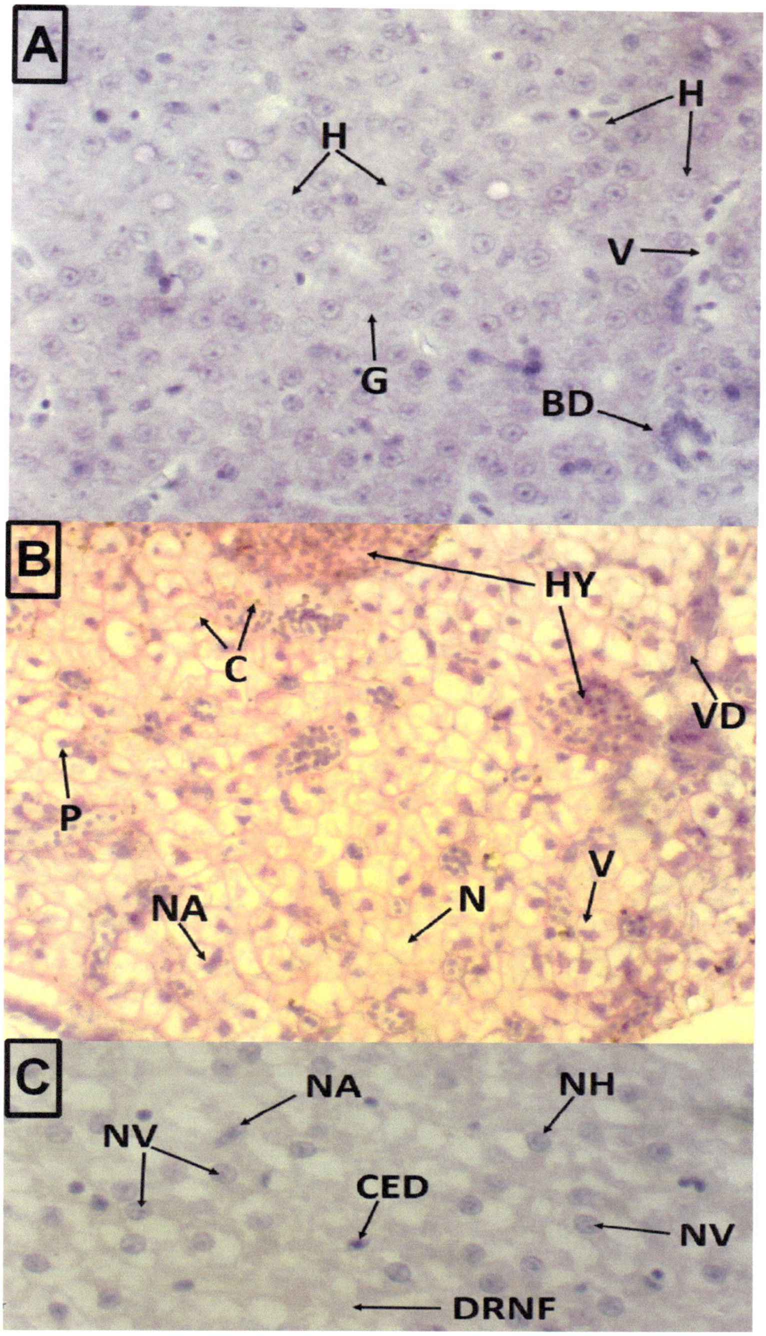

Figure 2.
Comparison between normal and changed liver tissues. (A) Healthy liver tissue, where H is the hepatocytes; V, blood vessels; BD, bile ducts; G, glycogen. (B) and (C) Changed liver tissue with typical histopathological changes, such as HY, hyperemia; V, vacuolization; P, pycnosis; C, cholestasis; N, necrosis; VD, vessel degeneration; NV, nucleus vacuolization; NA, nucleus atrophy; NH, nucleus hypertrophy; CED, cellular degeneration; DRNF, relative decrease of nuclei frequency (H&E, ×40).

by the Bowman capsule, while the tubules are surrounded by epithelial cells. Hematopoietic, interrenal, and chromaffin cells [7] are also observed in the interstice of the kidney.

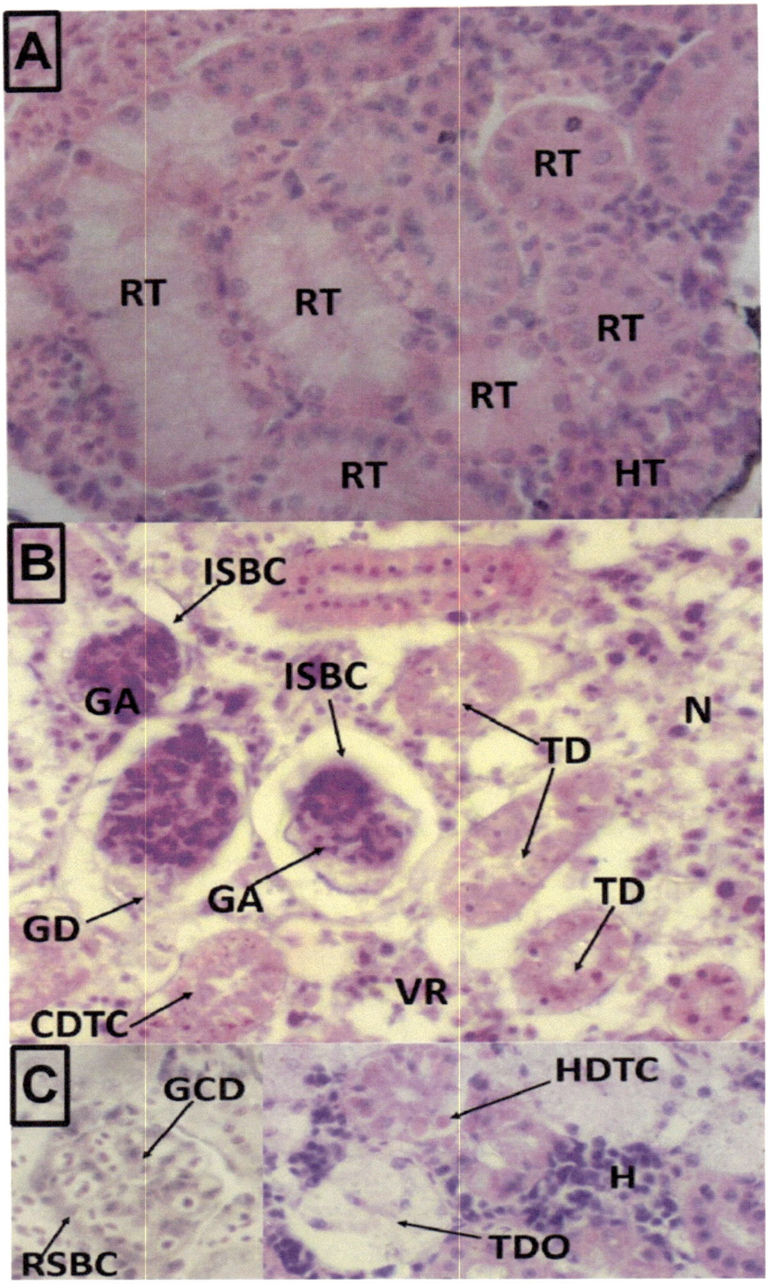

Figure 3.
Comparison between normal and changed kidney tissues. (A) Healthy kidney tissue, where RT is the renal tubules; HT, hematopoietic tissue. (B) Changed kidney tissue with typical histopathological changes, such as GA, glomerular atrophy; GD, glomerular degeneration; ISBC, increased space of the Bowman capsule; CDTC, cytoplasmatic degeneration of tubular cells; TD, tubular degeneration; VR, vessel rupture; N, necrosis. (C) Changed kidney tissue with GCD, glomerular capillaries dilation; RSBC, reduced space of the Bowman capsule; HDTC, hyaline degeneration of tubular cells; TDO, tubular disorganization; H, hyperemia (H&E, ×40).

The interrenal cells have an endocrine role functionally equivalent to the mammals' adrenal cortex and are accountable to synthesize cortisol in response to physiological stress. On the other hand, the chromaffin cells are functionally equivalent to the adrenal medulla and synthesize epinephrine and norepinephrine, which will act in the cardiac rhythm [7].

In contact with toxic compounds, the most frequent tissue alterations of the kidney are found in the tubules. The hypertrophy of tubule cells is an alteration caused by dryness of the epithelial cells surrounding the tubules, which is caused by alterations in the filtration of the kidney. Frequent structural tissue alterations in the tubular cells include tubular disorganization, tubular degeneration, and cytoplasmatic degeneration. According to Carvalho et al. [5], these tubular alterations found in the kidney of zebrafish can be caused indirectly by metabolic dysfunction caused by toxic compounds.

When tubular cells are functionally changed, hyaline degeneration can occur, evidenced by the occurrence of eosinophilic granules their cytoplasm [5]. Hyaline degeneration can be caused by reabsorption of protein compounds excessively synthesized by the glomeruli [33].

Toxic compounds can also affect the function of the kidney glomeruli. In some cases, this can cause glomerulus atrophy or degeneration evidenced by the increase in the Bowman capsule space. In other situations, dilation of the glomerulus' capillaries can occur, which is a mechanism to reduce tissue damage by increasing the blood flow to the area.

The reduction of the Bowman capsule space can compromise the renal filtration, while the over increased hyperemia can potentially induce rupture of blood vessels [5, 29]. Both of these tissue changes can result in kidney necrosis [33]. The tissue changes often observed in the kidney of zebrafish are shown in **Figure 3**.

3.4 Intestine

The intestine of zebrafish is formed by villi, surrounded by a mucous layer. In the center of these villi is the lamina propria, where defense cells are found. Along the villi, there are the mucus-producing goblet cells and the enterocytes, accountable of nutrient absorption in the epithelium; the enterocytes also have a role in the immune response and osmotic balance [5, 9, 27]. Exposure to toxic compounds can damage the intestinal mucosa and hamper the cellular development in this tissue, causing a disturbance in its physiology evidenced by histological changes [5, 33].

A typical feature of injury caused by noxious compounds in the intestine is inflammation in the lamina propria. Inflammation is characterized by leukocyte infiltration, mainly neutrophils, with a morphology similar to mammals (clear cytoplasm and multi-lobed nuclei). Other inflammatory cells of zebrafish are the lymphocytes and monocytes, also similar to those of mammals [7].

The infiltration of eosinophils in the tissue caused by inflammation corroborates to the increased hyperemia [5, 34]. When stained with hematoxylin and eosin, these cells have a deeper pink-colored cytoplasm and a rounded peripheral nucleus [7]. A defense mechanism to avoid injury caused by leukocyte infiltration in the villi is the separation of lamina propria, which reduces the contact between the inflammatory cells and the enterocytes.

Another feature observed in the enterocytes after exposure to highly toxic compounds is vacuolization, which can be accompanied by edema. This latter is often associated with degeneration of the muscle layer and the villi. These tissue changes hamper the process of nutrient absorption and often precede necrosis [5, 33]. In **Figure 4** the typical intestine structure and the main tissue changes cited in this section are shown.

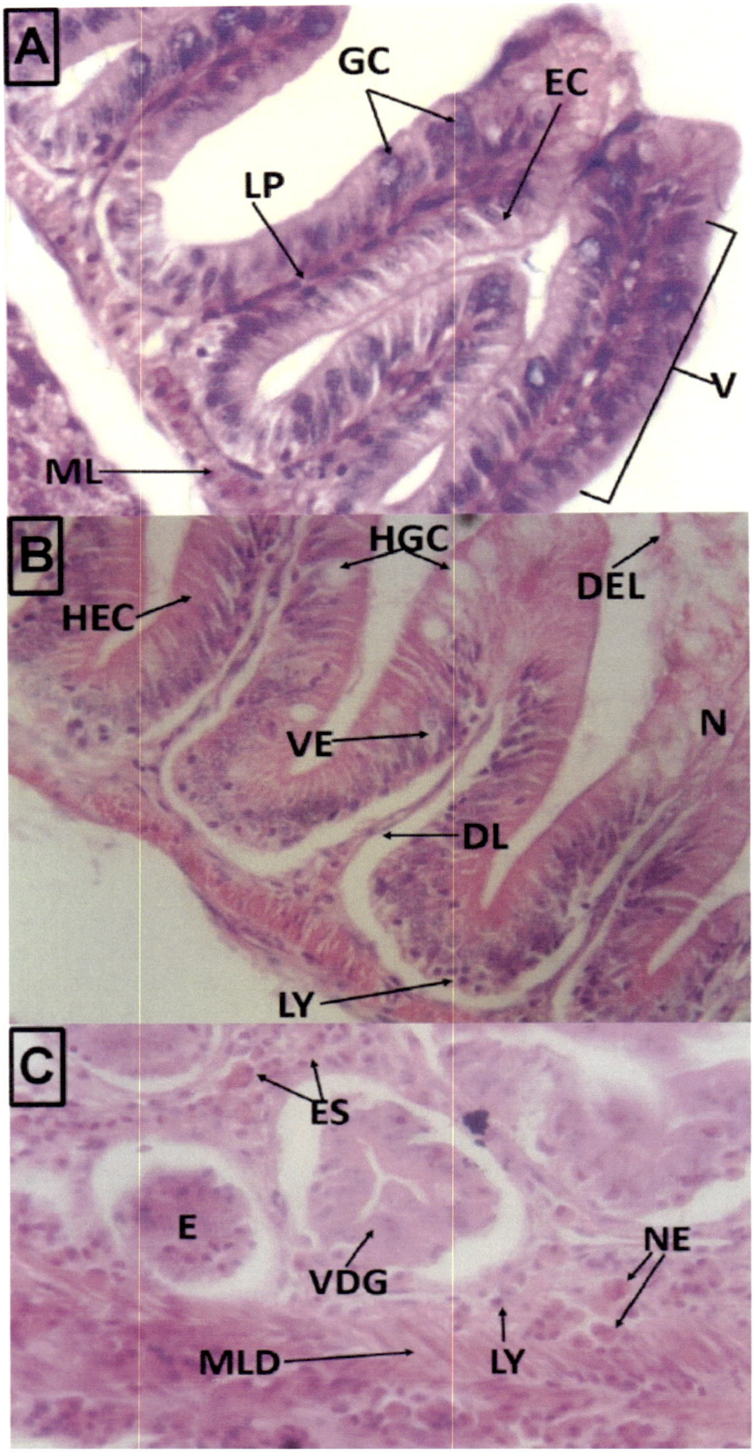

Figure 4.
Comparison between normal and changed intestine tissues. (A) Healthy intestine tissue, where V is the villi; LP, lamina propria; EC, enterocytes; GC, goblet cells; ML, muscle layer. (B) Changed intestine tissue with typical histopathological changes, such as HEC, hypertrophy of enterocytes; HGC, hyperplasia of goblet cells; VE, vacuolization of the enterocytes; DL, displacement of the lamina propria; DEL, detachment of the epithelium; LY, lymphocytes; N, necrosis. (C) Intestine lamina propria inflammation, with NE, neutrophils; LY, lymphocytes; ES, eosinophils; E, edema; VDG, villi degeneration; MLD, muscle layer degeneration (H&E, ×40).

4. Conclusion

This chapter, written by researchers of pharmaceutical and biological sciences, is intended for college students, postgraduation students, and researchers in the fields of biomedical science and related specialties. It is expected to aid researchers in the field of histopathology and toxicology to better understand the application of zebrafish in these areas. Relevant information about tissue changes are gathered caused by exposure to toxic agents in zebrafish and its potential application as a model in nonclinical toxicological studies. In this chapter previously unpublished pictures are presented that can serve as a primer for the study of healthy and changed tissues of gills, liver, kidney, and intestine of zebrafish.

Acknowledgements

The authors thank the Coordination for the Improvement of Higher Education Personnel (CAPES – Procad Amazônia Proc. 88887.200554/2018–2100) and National Council for Scientific and Technological Development (CNPq) - Proc. 402,332/2013–0.

Conflicts of interest

The author(s) declared no potential conflicts of interest with respect to the research, authorship, and/or publication of this chapter.

Author details

Raphaelle Sousa Borges[1,2], Arlindo César Matias Pereira[1,2], Gisele Custodio de Souza[1,2] and José Carlos Tavares Carvalho[1,2]*

1 Programa de Pós-graduação em Ciências Farmacêuticas, Departamento de Ciências Biológicas e da Saúde, Universidade Federal do Amapá, Macapá, Amapá, Brazil

2 Laboratório de Pesquisa em Fármacos, Curso de Farmácia, Departamento de Ciências Biológicas e da Saúde, Universidade Federal do Amapá, Macapá, Amapá, Brazil

*Address all correspondence to: farmacos@unifap.br

References

[1] Poon KL, Brand T. The zebrafish model system in cardiovascular research: A tiny fish with mighty prospects. Global Cardiology Science and Practice. 2013;**2013**(1):4

[2] dos Santos VF, Duarte JL, Pinho Fernandes C, Keita H, Rafael Rodríguez Amado J, Arturo Velázquez-Moyado J, et al. Use of zebrafish (*Danio rerio*) in experimental models for biological assay with natural products. African Journal of Pharmacy and Pharmacology. 2016;**10**(42):883-891

[3] Huang SY, Feng CW, Hung HC, Chakraborty C, Chen CH, Chen WF, et al. A novel zebrafish model to provide mechanistic insights into the inflammatory events in carrageenan-induced abdominal edema. PLoS One. 2014;**9**(8):e104414

[4] Howe K, Clark MD, Torroja CF, Torrance J, Berthelot C, Muffato M, et al. The zebrafish reference genome sequence and its relationship to the human genome. Nature. 2013;**496**(7446):498-503

[5] Carvalho JCT, Keita H, Santana GR, de Souza GC, dos Santos IVF, Amado JRR, et al. Effects of bothrops alternatus venom in zebrafish: A histopathological study. Inflammopharmacology. 2018 Feb 17;**26**(1):273-284. DOI: 10.1007/s10787-017-0362-z

[6] Heath AG. Water Pollution and Fish Physiology. Boca Raton: CRC Press; 2018. Available from: https://www.taylorfrancis.com/books/9781351404990

[7] Menke AL, Spitsbergen JM, Wolterbeek APM, Woutersen RA. Normal anatomy and histology of the adult zebrafish. Toxicologic Pathology. 2011;**39**(5):759-775

[8] Vliegenthart ADB, Tucker CS, Del Pozo J, Dear JW. Zebrafish as model organisms for studying drug-induced liver injury. British Journal of Clinical Pharmacology. 2014;**78**(6):1217-1227

[9] Borges RS, Keita H, Ortiz BLS, dos Santos Sampaio TI, Ferreira IM, Lima ES, et al. Anti-inflammatory activity of nanoemulsions of essential oil from *Rosmarinus officinalis* L.: in vitro and in zebrafish studies. Inflammopharmacology. 2018;**26**(4):1057-1080. DOI: 10.1007/s10787-017-0438-9

[10] Scholz S, Fischer S, Gündel U, Küster E, Luckenbach T, Voelker D. The zebrafish embryo model in environmental risk assessment—Applications beyond acute toxicity testing. Environmental Science and Pollution Research. 2008;**15**(5):394-404

[11] de Souza GC, Duarte JL, Fernandes CP, Velázquez-Moyado J, Navarrete A, JCT C. Obtainment and study of the toxicity of perillyl alcohol nanoemulsion on Zebrafish (*Danio rerio*). Journal of Nanomedicine Research. 2016;**4**(4):18-20. Available from: http://medcraveonline.com/JNMR/JNMR-04-00093.php

[12] Van Der Ven LTM, Van Den Brandhof EJ, Vos JH, Power DM, Wester PW. Effects of the antithyroid agent propylthiouracil in a partial life cycle assay with zebrafish. Environmental Science & Technology. 2006;**40**(1):74-81

[13] Velasco-Santamaría YM, Korsgaard B, Madsen SS, Bjerregaard P. Bezafibrate, a lipid-lowering pharmaceutical, as a potential endocrine disruptor in male zebrafish (*Danio rerio*). Aquatic Toxicology. 2011;**105**(1-2):107-118

[14] de Souza GC, Matias Pereira AC, Viana MD, Ferreira AM, da Silva IDR, de Oliveira MMR, et al. Acmella

oleracea (L) R. K. Jansen reproductive toxicity in zebrafish: An in vivo and in silico assessment. Evidence-based Complementary and Alternative Medicine. 2019;**2019**:1-19

[15] Cheepurupalli L, Raman T, Rathore SS, Ramakrishnan J. Bioactive molecule from *streptomyces* sp. mitigates MDR *Klebsiella pneumoniae* in zebrafish infection model. Frontiers in Microbiology. 2017;**8**:1-15

[16] Jianjie C, Wenjuan X, Jinling C, Jie S, Ruhui J, Meiyan L. Fluoride caused thyroid endocrine disruption in male zebrafish (*Danio rerio*). Aquatic Toxicology. 2016;**171**:48-58

[17] Barillet S, Larno V, Floriani M, Devaux A, Adam-Guillermin C. Ultrastructural effects on gill, muscle, and gonadal tissues induced in zebrafish (*Danio rerio*) by a waterborne uranium exposure. Aquatic Toxicology. 2010;**100**(3):295-302. DOI: 10.1016/j.aquatox.2010.08.002

[18] Hou LP, Yang Y, Shu H, Ying GG, Zhao JL, Chen YB, et al. Changes in histopathology, enzyme activities, and the expression of relevant genes in zebrafish (*Danio rerio*) following long-term exposure to environmental levels of thallium. Bulletin of Environmental Contamination and Toxicology. 2017;**99**(5):574-581. DOI: 10.1007/s00128-017-2176-5

[19] Hussainzada N, Lewis JA, Baer CE, Ippolito DL, Jackson DA, Stallings JD. Whole adult organism transcriptional profiling of acute metal exposures in male zebrafish. BMC Pharmacology and Toxicology. 2014;**15**(1):1-15

[20] Qian L, Zhang J, Chen X, Qi S, Wu P, Wang C, et al. Toxic effects of boscalid in adult zebrafish (*Danio rerio*) on carbohydrate and lipid metabolism. Environmental Pollution. 2019;**247**:775-782. DOI: 10.1016/j.envpol.2019.01.054

[21] Liu C, Su G, Giesy JP, Letcher RJ, Li G, Agrawal I, et al. Acute exposure to tris(1,3-dichloro-2-propyl) phosphate (TDCIPP) causes hepatic inflammation and leads to hepatotoxicity in zebrafish. Scientific Reports. 2016;**6**:1-11. DOI: 10.1038/srep19045

[22] Madureira TV, Rocha MJ, Cruzeiro C, Rodrigues I, Monteiro RAF, Rocha E. The toxicity potential of pharmaceuticals found in the Douro River estuary (Portugal): Evaluation of impacts on fish liver, by histopathology, stereology, vitellogenin and CYP1A immunohistochemistry, after sub-acute exposures of the zebrafish model. Environmental Toxicology and Pharmacology. 2012;**34**(1):34-45. DOI: 10.1016/j.etap.2012.02.007

[23] Du Y, Shi X, Liu C, Yu K, Zhou B. Chronic effects of water-borne PFOS exposure on growth, survival and hepatotoxicity in zebrafish: A partial life-cycle test. Chemosphere. 2009;**74**(5):723-729. DOI: 10.1016/j.chemosphere.2008.09.075

[24] Osborne OJ, Lin S, Chang CH, Ji Z, Yu X, Wang X, et al. Organ-specific and size-dependent Ag nanoparticle toxicity in gills and intestines of adult zebrafish. ACS Nano. 2015;**9**(10):9573-9584

[25] Renieri EA, Sfakianakis DG, Alegakis AA, Safenkova IV, Buha A, Matović V, et al. Nonlinear responses to waterborne cadmium exposure in zebrafish. An in vivo study. Environmental Research. 2017;**157**:173-181

[26] Vesna P, Mitrovic-Tutundzic V. Fish gills as a monitor of sublethal and chronic effects of pollution. In: Sublethal and Chronic Effects of Pollutants on Freshwater Fish. Oxford: Fishing News Books; 1994. pp. 339-352

[27] Holden JA, Lester J, JLM L. The zebrafish: Atlas of macroscopic and microscopic anatomy. Cambridge, UK: Cambridge University Press;

2012;**86**:147. ISBN: (Paperback) 978-1107621343

[28] Campagna AF, Fracacio R, Rodrigues BK, Eler MN, Fenerich-Verani N, Espindola ELG. Effects of the copper in the survival, growth and gill morphology of *Danio rerio* (Cypriniformes, Cyprinidae). Acta Limnologica Brasiliensia. 2008;**20**(3):253-259. Available from: papers2://publication/uuid/31BDFF0B-22B1-425D-BD00-A272492CFD27

[29] Meletti PC. Avaliação da degradação ambiental por meio de testes de toxicidade com sedimento e de análises histopatológicas em peixes. São Carlos: Universidade de São Paulo; 2016. Available from: http://www.teses.usp.br/teses/disponiveis/18/18139/tde-02082016-121212/

[30] Mazon AF, Cerqueira CCC, Fernandes MN. Gill cellular changes induced by copper exposure in the south American tropical freshwater fish *Prochilodus scrofa*. Environmental Research. 2002;**88**(1):52-63

[31] Rezende KFO, Santos RM, Borges JCS, Salvo LM, Da Silva JRMHC. Histopathological and genotoxic effects of pollution on Nile tilapia (*Oreochromis niloticus*, Linnaeus, 1758) in the Billings reservoir (Brazil). Toxicology Mechanisms and Methods. 2014;**24**(6):404-411

[32] Van Den Heuvel MR, Power M, Richards J, MacKinnon M, Dixon DG. Disease and gill lesions in yellow perch (*Perca flavescens*) exposed to oil sands mining-associated waters. Ecotoxicology and Environmental Safety. 2000;**46**(3):334-341

[33] Caspers H. An atlas of fish histology. Normal and pathological features. In: Hibiya T, editor. International Review of Hydrobiology. Vol. 69. Stuttgart/New York: John Wiley and Sons; 1984. pp. 406-406. DOI: 10.1002/iroh.19840690307

[34] Roberts RJ, Ellis AE. The anatomy and physiology of Teleosts. In: Fish Pathology. 4th ed. 2012. pp. 17-61